Sexual Interactions and HIV Risk

Social Aspects of AIDS
Series Editor: Peter Aggleton
Institute of Education, University of London

Editorial Advisory Board

Sexual Interactions and HIV Risk

New Conceptual Perspectives in European Research

Edited by

Luc Van Campenhoudt, Mitchell Cohen,
Gustavo Guizzardi, Dominique Hausser

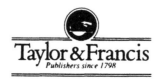

Taylor & Francis
Publishers since 1798

First published 1997
By Taylor & Francis
2 Park Square, Milton Park, Abingdon, Oxon, OX14 4RN
270 Madison Ave, New York NY 10016

Transferred to Digital Printing 2006

A Catalogue Record for this book is available from the British Library

ISBN 0 7484 0345 0
ISBN 0 7484 0346 9 (pbk)

Library of Congress Cataloging-in-Publication Data are available on request

Series cover design by Barking Dog Art
Additional artwork by Hyberts Design & Type

Typeset in 10/12 pt Baskerville
by Graphicraft Typesetters Limited, Hong Kong

Publisher's Note
The publisher has gone to great lengths to ensure the quality of this reprint but points out that some imperfections in the original may be apparent

Contents

Contents

List of Figures and Tables

Figures

Tables

Series Editor's Preface

Worldwide, the most frequent means by which HIV is transmitted is through unprotected vaginal or anal sex. Research into the nature of sexual interaction is therefore of the utmost importance for the development of interventions to prevent and interrupt transmission. Yet many existing frameworks by which sexual interaction are analysed and 'made sense' of are overly simple to say the least, positing too direct a relationship between knowledge, beliefs and behaviour, for example, or marginalizing the impact of structural and environmental factors as determinants of human sexual behaviour.

Sexual Interactions and HIV Risk seeks to remedy some of these deficiencies, and reports on work carried out as part of a major European Concerted Action on sexual behaviour and the risks of HIV infection. Its authors all participated in this action, developing in the process new ways of understanding the various dimensions of sexual relationships, including the role of power, emotion, meaning, time and risk-taking, among other variables, in structuring sexual interaction, and in affecting HIV-related risks. Along with its companion text *Sexual Behaviour and HIV/AIDS in Europe* (Hubert, Bajos and Sandfort (Eds), Taylor & Francis, forthcoming), this book will undoubtedly serve as an important reference point for years to come.

Peter Aggleton

Introduction

Research into HIV/AIDS risk-related behaviour calls for more theories, but at the same time investigators and prevention practitioners are wary of theories. Both attitudes are well-founded. Without theories, there is little hope of contributing to a larger picture the reasons for changing or maintaining safer or unsafe sexual practices. On the other hand, theorizing is often perceived as resulting from arbitrariness and prejudices. It may seem murky and uselessly complicated, so that in the final analysis it no longer has any practical worth. What is more, the social sciences in particular suffer from the tendency to formulate numerous competing theories that reject each other. Efforts to develop theories seem to go off in all directions, without any clear order. In the end, all theoretical work loses some of its credibility. This volume was thus conceived in a specific and unusual way, in terms of both its content and the approach taken, in order to meet these very problems.

In this book, European researchers offer new conceptual frameworks that focus on interactions between partners and among social networks and suggest their application to HIV/AIDS prevention programs. The book also offers a critique of the individual-oriented perspectives that have been the dominant basis for research and prevention programs over the past decade. While individual characteristics do exert influence over behaviour, it is a contention of this volume that they become salient only in the interactions between partners and among peers, in a particular socio-cultural context.

We have attempted to develop a clear organization in this book that provides discussion of the complementary themes and contradictions of the authors. We believe the book is of use both theoretically and practically, and that it moves toward structuring an emerging scientific field of interaction-oriented perspectives of sexual behaviour. The book is organized in four sections, each with an introduction, original contributions and a summary and discussion chapter. The first section, Sexual Interaction and HIV Risk-related Behaviour, presents several theoretical perspectives that focus on the interaction processes. The introduction to Section I and the discussion in Chapter 4 present the main landmarks that will be used to structure the theoretical field throughout the remainder of the book. Section II, From Individual to Interaction, criticizes individual-oriented theories as its starting point, and shows how the findings of research inspired by such theories both contradict and complement interaction-based research. It ends with a discussion of the rationality of behaviour. Section III, Interaction and its Socio-cultural Context, studies the links between macro- and micro-social processes. In Chapter 10 the theoretical and operational links between interaction-oriented, individual-oriented and social and cultural contexts are conceptualized. Section IV, From Theory to Prevention, focuses on how the policymakers and prevention providers can incorporate interaction-oriented concepts into prevention programs. It discusses the process of creating, diffusing, and enforcing safer sexual norms given the contradictions between preventive messages and the ideologies that underlie them. Section IV emphasizes the importance of building prevention programs based on the priorities of those who are the targets of prevention programs and planning when and what types of prevention are appropriate. It reinforces the overall message of the book that it is time to move from individual-oriented prevention based on the linear correlations between safer sex and knowledge, attitude, beliefs and behavioural factors. The alternative is prevention based on understanding the meaning and dynamics of these factors in specific situations where sex is the outcome of interactions between partners and among social networks. Also included is a glossary of the main concepts that underlie several chapters of this book.

The Process

The book is an outgrowth of a European Concerted Action on Sexual Behaviour and Risks of HIV Infection.[1] The process of the Concerted Action led to the diversified viewpoints and international collaborations reflected in this volume. In a first meeting in Portugal in November 1991, an agreement was reached among the 35 participants from 12 countries that the Concerted Action would undertake two separate activities: 1) an investigation of new conceptual perspectives from a European viewpoint; and 2) a comparison of empirical data about sexual behaviour and the risk of HIV from general population studies throughout Europe. This book is the outcome of the first activity. A comparative analysis of the main surveys on sexual behaviour and HIV risk carried out recently in Europe will be published as another book, *Sexual Behaviour and HIV/AIDS in Europe*, edited by Michel Hubert, Nathalie Bajos and Theo Sandfort, in this same series (*Social Aspects of AIDS*). The initial input for this book was a series of original texts (what we call the basic texts) written by at least two investigators from different countries. They included researchers from Belgium, France, Germany, Great Britain, Greece, Italy, the Netherlands and Switzerland each with different backgrounds and theoretical references. Some of the authors already knew each other, the rest met each other during the preparatory meetings thanks to the Concerted Action. A second phase of activity for this book involved systematic comparison of the texts prepared by different authors and a discussion among the authors in a three-day workshop in Brussels in September 1993. The workshop was organized around the following five themes:

1 the conceptualization of interactions;
2 the rationality or non-rationality of individuals;
3 normative tensions;
4 the limits and scope of explanation; and
5 prevention.

This type of joint working arrangement was chosen to facilitate the comparison between different theories and even, in some of the texts, different fields, and also to create and consolidate a European scientific community with regard to these problems. The structuring of a field of research is indeed indissociable from the structuring of a community of researchers who acquire the ability and habit of working together. Finally, the introductions and some summary chapters were written after the meetings to facilitate the linking of the sections and the overall structuring of interaction-oriented frameworks of HIV/AIDS risk-related sexual behaviour. This book is thus the result of collective work, even if each chapter reflects solely its authors' opinions and ethical point of view.

Reader's Guide

The book may be read in three ways. The first way consists of reading each basic text for itself (Chapters 1, 2, 3, 5, 6, 8, 9 and 11). Apart from the summaries and discussion chapters, these chapters can stand on their own merits. The second way consists in focusing on one or more of the four main sections of the book. Each of these sections consists of an introduction, two or three basic texts plus a summary and discussion. The third way is to follow the structuring of the theoretical field of HIV/AIDS risk-related behaviour based on interactions. In this case, the introductions to the four different parts become the road map for the book, for they link and weave together the concepts that emerge from each chapter and section.

The function of this effort is both theoretical and heuristic; theoretical because it makes it possible to situate each perspective within a field of theories and heuristic because it proposes an ordered set of hypotheses and conceptual resources to be used by the reader for future research or prevention work.

Acknowledgments

No such undertaking is complete without acknowledging the contributions of all those involved in the effort. The editors were the driving forces behind this endeavour, in which dialogue and debate between themselves and with the authors were constant processes. The authors contributed much time and effort and the editors gratefully acknowledge their involvement in the workshops, revisions on their texts and their willingness to accept certain modifications to ensure the overall consistency of the book. The authors exhibited a remarkable research spirit, marked by their openness to each others' ideas, to discussion and to calling ideas into question.

Translating into English and editing a set of texts from several different countries and disciplines has been a challenge. The editors are thus extremely grateful for the translations and grammar and reference checks done by Gaby Leyden, Anne Heynderyckx, Theodore Trefon and Gaïl Fagen. A considerable part of the final editing was done by Mitchell Cohen and we owe a debt of gratitude to the government of the Brussels Region for his support through a grant under its Research in Brussels Programme.

Nothing, however, would have been possible without the constant help of the Concerted Action's Coordinating Unit, especially that of Michel Hubert, the project leader, and Josette Jamet, its secretariat incarnate.[1] Finally, the confidence and constant support of the Commission of the European Communities representatives involved in the Biomedical and Health Research Programme (BIOMED) helped us immensely. We should like to express our particular gratitude to the late Mr G. Everard, to Dr M.C. Razquin, and, above all, to Dr A.E. Baert, Head of the Medical Research Unit at the European Commission (DG XII-E-4), who supported our project from the start.

Note

1 The purpose of this Concerted Action – a four-year research project – which was coordinated by the *Centre d'études sociologiques* of *Facultés universitaires Saint-Louis*, (Project Leader: Michel Hubert) in Brussels, was to contribute to the development of a European scientific community dealing with the study of sexual behaviour and attitudes to HIV risk.

Section I

Sexual Interaction and Risk-related Behaviour

Introduction

The main aim of this section is to conceptualize interactions between sexual partners and suggest prospects for prevention based on partner interactions within the context of cultural norms. Chapter 1 by Ferrand and Snijders, explains how social networks and norms are related to sexual behaviour. The relationship between the partners is viewed as part of a social network. In Chapter 2, Ahlemeyer applies systems theory from a sociological perspective to different intimate communication patterns. His co-author Ludwig shows how recent contributions from cognitive and social psychological theories help in understanding sexual behaviour that results from the interactions between partners. In Chapter 3, Bastard, Cardia-Vonèche, Peto and Van Campenhoudt draw from different sociological models in describing several social factors related to sexual behaviour. In the last chapter of this section, Van Campenhoudt and Cohen explore the forms of causality used by the preceding authors and suggest implications for explaining sexual behaviour related to the risk of HIV infection. Referring to the broad concept of causality, Van Campenhoudt and Cohen first discuss the differences between the epistemological, theoretical and methodological characteristics used by the authors to explain sexual behaviour. They then review how the different perspectives deal with various dimensions of sexual relationships: the situation, time, meaning, power, sexuality, emotion and risk taking.

The investigation of interaction-oriented behaviour is necessary, particularly given the poor track record of individual-based models of behaviour change. However, we admit from the start that no single perspective, despite its pertinence and sophistication, can fully explain sexual behaviour. What is more, all behavioural theories are contingent on basic premises that are likely to be modified as the environment and fields of application change. In beginning any research project investigators usually confine themselves to studying a limited range of social phenomena. In evaluating the explanatory value of different perspectives, one must consider what specific and limited contribution each theory makes to an understanding of HIV-related risk behaviour. For example: What does a perspective reveal and elucidate and what does it not allow one to study? What does it add that differs from or expands upon the contributions of other perspectives? What criteria of validity must be applied to the theory, given its epistemological foundations? Once this is done, it is possible to structure these perspectives into a scientific field with a practical purpose such as preventing HIV infection and AIDS.

However, structuring a scientific field will not, in itself, lead to an all-encompassing, conciliatory *megaperspective* in which contradictions between approaches are resolved and all debate avoided. If that were the case, each perspective would lose its own power to elucidate reality! On the contrary, an effort must be made to challenge the internal consistency of each perspective and take each perspective to its logical limits.

The search for causality has fermented considerable debate in the social sciences, where deterministic explanations and linear cause-and-effect relationships have dominated the models used to predict sexual behaviour. We argue in this book for causal explanations with a broader meaning than a simple deterministic blueprint. Instead, we think causality should mean a reconstitution of the *process* that leads from the causes of sexual behaviour to the observed sexual behaviour, even to the genesis of the sexual behaviour. The cause then becomes 'that which, *in one way or another*, belongs to the constitution of the phenomenon or, in other words, is revealed as a moment of the phenomenalisation' (Ladrière, 1994). When taken in this broad sense, causality can be considered the tool for scientific explanation.

In discussing the first three chapters in this section, Van Campenhoudt and Cohen make the distinction between formal and material causes. As an illustration of this distinction, Franck (1994), uses the analogy of the chess game. The formal cause is like the rules of the game that must be understood if one is to play or make useful observations about the game. However, these rules do not enable one to foresee the actual course of the game or how it will end. They cannot be used to reconstitute the phenomenon's actual genesis. When researchers rely on formal causes only, they lock themselves in a purely deterministic explanation of the phenomena. This sheds light on the *whys* and defines a field of possibilities, but does not explain the phenomena. To know the outcome of the game one must also know the actual conditions of the game, such as the adversaries' strengths, the climate of the game, whether the adversaries will react cautiously or boldly to each others' moves, the place the game occupies in the history of their matches, etc. The material cause accounts for the actual circumstances in which the system functions. The material cause enables us to explain *how*, in line with various circumstances and chains of actual events, a specific phenomenon, such as a behaviour change in response to the risk of AIDS, actually came about.

The systems approach espoused by Ahlemeyer and the social network theory presented by Ferrand and Snijders place more emphasis on formal causality, whereas other authors give more weight to material causality. So, from a systemic sociology standpoint, Ahlemeyer's text must be judged on the basis of its ability to define the field of sexual behaviour related to HIV/ AIDS risk and provide probabilities for the various sexual behaviours under study. In contrast, Bastard and Ludwig focus more on material causes. In their view, sexual behaviour is the result of a chain of actual circumstances. Their approach should be evaluated by how well it accounts for what actually happens. Indeed, this representation of phenomena also allows for causal processes and entails a theoretical construction that includes a conceptualization of the categories of events and circumstances to be considered (for example, the partners' positions in their life cycles or the phases of their relationship) and hypotheses concerning the influences of these events. If it is possible to speak about this in terms of description, we are thus dealing with a description that is built upon theory.

In Chapter 4, Van Campenhoudt and Cohen not only discuss the epistemological perspectives of the different approaches, but also explore the theoretical perspectives presented by the different authors. They search for sets of concepts and hypotheses which explain sexual behaviours related to HIV/AIDS risk. Specific concepts and hypotheses are key to each perspective; they also structure the entire perspective. The reader may find the discussion in Chapter 4 abstract, yet it starts the process of critically examining the different perspectives presented in the book. We believe it serves to present several criteria for comparing the various perspectives, restricts the criticism of perspectives based on misunderstandings, and opens debate regarding their assumptions and utility.

We understand that each chapter is independently valuable and may be read without any reference to this synthesis. Given this brief introduction, we hope the reader will tackle the following three core chapters of this section and then read Chapter 4, which presents a structure that facilitates comparison of the perspectives offered by the different authors.

References

FRANCK, R. (1994) *Faut-il chercher aux causes une raison? L'explication causale dans les sciences humaines,* Paris: Institut interdisciplinaire d'études épistémologiques.

LADRIÈRE, J. (1994) 'La causalité dans les sciences de la nature et dans les sciences humaines', in Franck, R. *Faut-il chercher aux causes une raison? L'explication causale dans les sciences humaines,* Paris: Institut interdisciplinaire d'études épistémologiques, pp. 248–74.

Chapter 1

Social Networks and Normative Tensions

Alexis Ferrand and Tom A.B. Snijders

Introduction

The body is our fundamental, primary environment. It offers us pleasure and pain. Sexual activities usually induce pleasure, but they can also induce illness and pain. The basic terms of the individualistic approach to health-oriented sexual behaviour suggest that: a) human beings are our secondary environment, and b) they can offer different kinds of physical and non-physical pleasure and pain because of who they are and how we are related to them. Sexual relations provide the most enjoyable and rewarding pleasures.

This chapter aims to transcend this individualistic approach and stress the relational dimension of sexual life from a sociological perspective. First we move from individual sexual behaviours to interpersonal-oriented sexual behaviour. Like all personal relations, sexual relations are embedded in personal networks. The relational perspective on sexual behaviour makes it necessary to understand how personal networks are formed and maintained and which functions they can fulfil. Among these functions we emphasize the production and reinforcement of collective norms of sexual behaviour, conditioned by specific properties of networks.

Sexual Life as Relational Processes

The most characteristic feature of sexual life is the impulse, feeling, affectivity between persons. Sexual life is made of links between pairs (or larger groups) of persons. These links exist at several levels: physical contact, language, and other types of interaction – including pure fantasy. Nobody can contest the general approach to analysing individual sex lives that takes the orientation of ego (the focal actor) toward alters (possible partners) in terms of mono/ pluri-partnership, homo/heterosexual orientation, self-erotization (as a retreat from the encountering of alter), and so on, into account.

Much research into sexual behaviour is based (often implicitly) on the paradigm of an actor trying to obtain sexual satisfaction from an inert environment. Within this paradigm, sexual interactions are explained mainly by the psychological and sociological backgrounds of separate individuals and the constraints implied by these backgrounds. Actors are assumed to pick more or less rewarding sexual partners as objects of their conscious and unconscious strategies. Such separately considered individuals are designated in this chapter as *focal actors*. This paradigm, however, raises the following theoretical problem: If the focal actors have a diverse set of characteristics which influence their strategies and actions, why are the sexual partners' properties defined simply in very broad, rough terms (such as gender, age, social and marital status)?

A relational theory of sexuality re-introduces into its approach the symmetry between ego and alter. Moreover, such a theory recognizes that the behaviour of actors (or partners) is not only restricted by the social context, but simultaneously influences and shapes the social context. All of us are egos to ourselves; to others we are alters as well as components of the social context. An example of the last aspect is that everybody has a role of upholding social norms, a role which may be fulfilled in strict, loose, deviant or other manners. The social environment, therefore, is not inert but in dynamic interaction with individuals. Such a relational theory of sexuality is complex. We prefer it because it has a better logical correspondence to the phenomena of sexual behaviour, because we hope it is also empirically more powerful, but not because it is more simple. This relational paradigm is grounded on a few basic postulates given below.

Postulate 1: Dyadic nature of sexuality: Sexuality is defined from the specific point of view of interactions between actors, with a focus on pairwise (dyadic) interactions. The object of the theory is the variety of processes by which social interpersonal relations are sexualized. These various sexualization processes are a specific domain in the broad field of interpersonal relations. Thus, the theoretical frame is partly the general frame of interpersonal relations and partly specific to sexual behaviour.

Postulate 2: Anticipation of alter's reactions: Any relation is viewed as a sequence of interactions. Dyadic interactions are a specific kind of behaviour in which an individual (*ego*) acts on the basis of the expected and perceived answers of another individual (*alter*). Expectations are also based on contextual social knowledge, norms, personal experiences and subjective expectations. Interactions involve reciprocal attempts at adjusting both actors' expectations and behaviours.

Postulate 3: Bargaining and change: Implicit or explicit bargaining allows actors to define what is at the present moment relevant for their relationship. Any relation is a process, and may be stable over a long period or change rapidly. Different kinds of sexualization are steps in a whole relational process. They appear at certain moments, they can be transformed into different relational behaviour, and they can end.

Postulate 4: Embeddedness of relations in networks: For each actor, any relation is an element in his or her system of interpersonal relationships, the so-called ego network. A relation links two actors and simultaneously takes part in the composition and structure of the two relational systems of the actors involved. In addition, other people can observe part of the relational behaviour of the two actors. This observation is incomplete and often distorted, but may influence the two actors as well as other persons.

Postulate 5: Flexibility of norms and values: Social norms and socially determined expectations are not rigid. Individuals and social groups can and do adjust their norms and expectations to their preferences, constraints, and the information available to them. This holds also for norms and expectations that have a bearing on the ways in which relationships are sexualized. For example, when in many western countries the pill became available in the 1960s as a convenient new method of contraception, this implied a change in restrictions on sexual relations and the consequences of unprotected sexual intercourse. This led to important changes in behaviour and, eventually, norms and expectations. The information that may initiate or facilitate changing norms and expectations can be of a public nature (e.g., generally available knowledge about the reliability of contraceptive methods) but can also be formed of personal experiences (e.g., having undergone an abortion).

Bargaining (Postulate 3) and embeddedness (Postulate 4) imply a theoretical ambiguity of each relation, which must be understood partly as a specific relational process with its own history and partly as an element in both egos' network structures. Clearly, at present, there does not exist a complete and explicit theory that integrates this ambiguity. Instead, the ambiguity is managed through partial, middle-range propositions (based on the psychosociology of relational processes and the sociology of network structure).

It is impossible to engage here in a thorough discussion of the implications and developments of these general postulates. We shall thus mention five specific aspects.

1)   Sexualization covers the whole range of interactions by which a relation can provide affective, physical, and social rewards defined by actors as sexual: from platonic *rendezvous* to hard intercourse. Sexualization as a process, as a sequence of different kinds of interactions, is a central issue for the prevention of health-endangering behaviour. For example, often regardless of any new information about each other, sexual partners may abandon condom use simply because their relationship, by its own existence, generates new conditions for self-continuation. The chance of HIV transmission through sexual contacts creates a contradiction between the durability of the objective risk attached to an infected person, and the dynamics of any interpersonal love relation. Rapidly evolving reciprocal trust impedes the partners' ability to maintain safe sex conditions (Peto *et al.*, 1992). Similarly, actors who meet socially after a short

separation often suppose they know each other's sex life and therefore don't have to take precautions when they engage in a sexual relationship. Many people assume that their own social circle is clean; social proximity is thus often seen as a guarantee of safety. This illustrates again how the new situation created by the HIV epidemic has upset the balance between emotions, cognitions, and behaviour that regulates the sexualization of social relations.

2)   A study of sexuality along these lines cannot be based merely on cross-sections of behaviour, but must take into account the development of inter-action processes. As it is already difficult to propose a robust typology of instantaneous sexual behaviour, the idea of studying the relational process, thereby identifying successive changes in relationships, seems enormously complex and diverse. But we have to keep in mind that a prevention-oriented analysis is possible only on the basis of the study of relational processes, were it only because it is necessary to capture the change from the unsafe to safe condition and from safe to unsafe.

3)   As a consequence, actors do not have *a* behaviour. They may have several behaviours in a given relation through time and, at the same time, in different relations as a result of specific bargaining with different partners.

4)   It follows from Postulate 4 (embeddedness) that the affective, symbolic, and social demands made by actors in a sexual relationship depend also on actual and expected rewards in other possible sexual relations; and, more broadly, in other significant interpersonal ties. For example, the routinization of leisure life and socializing can lead to exceptional sexual relations' focusing on demands for change, uncertainty, and risk. Such compensation is one of many possible patterns.

5)   Because individuals are embedded in social networks (Postulates 4) and social norms are not rigid (Postulate 5), there is a feedback between actors' behaviour in a social system, mediated by a change of norms. When individuals perceive changes in sexualization patterns in the behaviour of others in their personal network, this will change their expectations and norms, which will in turn change their behaviour; this changed behaviour will feed back to and influence the behaviour of the others in their personal network.

The Influence of Sociability on Sexuality

Effects of Social Context on Sociability

Since sexual relationships are a specific subset of interpersonal relations, we present some relevant general traits of sociability, i.e., of the general ways in which people relate to one another. Two important aspects of the social context are: the composition of the wider social surroundings; and the social network, i.e., the network in which ego's social network is embedded. The mass media plays a major role in disseminating information from the wider social environment, such as information about the prevalence of sexually transmitted diseases. The media provides a base value for the individual's estimates of the risks associated with various sexual activities. The social network may be regarded as the carrier of norms about behaviour and of more specific information about individuals infected with sexually transmitted diseases, etc.

Demographic Structure of a Community and Ties between Individuals

Who meets whom? Who maintains some sort of interpersonal relationship with whom? These are two of the more general questions about sociability. An important aspect is the social hierarchy of status: how do attributes, such as the domains of professional occupation or social prestige, have an influence on interpersonalities? A classical postulate is that everybody prefers to meet another ego, someone of the same status with characteristics similar to one's own; such a tendency is called *homophily*. This postulate is confirmed in many empirical studies. However, the existence of a relation presupposes that actors have a chance to meet. Peter Blau has shown that this chance depends upon the social composition of the local community: 'our macrosociological objective is to examine how patterns of social relations in a community are affected by the social environment because the other people in their environment determine the options people have in establishing social relations' (Blau and Schwartz, 1984). The demographic composition of the population imposes limits on interpersonal choice, regardless of the value-orientations and preferences that individuals may have. The merit of such an analysis is to define statistical objective boundaries to personal choice; it is of little value to try to explain why so few people have good friends or lovers from a local minority if a high proportion of love-relationships with people in this minority is simply statistically impossible. An interesting study in this respect is Morris (1993), where the spread of a disease is modelled while taking into account sizes of sub-populations and differential contact rates between members of sub-populations.

Normative Differentiation and Overlapping of Social Fields in a Community

The cultural differentiation of the local community can also influence sociability. Cultural differentiation supposes that specific religious orientations, leisure activities, artistic trends, or modes of sexual behaviour have a sufficient number of supporters to reach a minimum level of collective institutional-ization through clubs, meeting places, social events, specialized shops, etc. The process of differentiation implies the emergence of various 'moral milieux' (to put it in the terms of Park) and contributes to the diversity of the urban way of life in the community (Gans, 1962).

The effect of cultural differentiation of the city is that a greater differ-ence between personal networks is possible. Fischer (1982) has shown that this effect is mediated by personal involvement: 'City life seems to aid people in finding other people who share their "most important" interest, but not in finding those who share lesser interests.' Those people involved in any kind of marginal sexual life have a higher chance of finding relational support and contextual legitimation of their behaviour in differentiated communities than in homogeneous communities. The question here is not the structure of the market of potential partners, as in Blau's perspective, but the emergence of social circles or contexts in which particular activities and relationships can be legitimized even if they are marginal or disapproved of by the silent majority. Thus cultural differentiation does not have a systematic effect on the composition of personal networks.

Another structural property of a community is the socio-spatial pattern of the activities that constitute specific social fields and offer opportunities to meet people. Locations of jobs, housing, shopping areas, leisure places can be separated (this is the typical pattern of modern *urban functional zoning*) or overlapping, which is a pattern found in the neighbourhoods of old Euro-pean towns or in some ghettos where residential, economic, and symbolic activities are clustered in the same place. If the cultural differentiation of the community allows the legitimation of different kinds of behaviour and pat-terns of relationships, the way in which that differentiation occurs does not determine directly the kind of social life one can have, but offers differential opportunities to get involved with others in various normative contexts or in a unique normatively homogeneous milieu. Such a differentiated community will also offer opportunities to choose between either dense interconnected or loosely knit segmented sets of interpersonal relations and contacts. Some consequences of these various opportunities will be presented below.

Mass Communication and Network Effects

Information and knowledge are disseminated through educational activities and mass media. Today, most people in modern countries have been in-formed about risks of transmission of AIDS. In several countries the risks of HIV infection are now covered in high school biology classes. What is the effect of such information on behaviour? This effect seems to be variable and often weak. Clearly, if networks of interpersonal relations affect how people react to the existence of the AIDS epidemic, it is not through their purely cognitive content.

Networks mediate information transmission in various ways. First, people make decisions about suggestions made in the public media because they are influenced by leaders or innovators. In the hypothesis of the 'two-step flow', the effect of a message is more powerful when the message is relayed by a 'local' opinion leader (Katz and Lazarsfeld, 1955). More broadly speaking, people seek differential advice from different persons in their social surroundings depending on the kind of decisions they have to make. The speed with which an innovation is adopted depends on the number and the type of interpersonal links people have that are related to the field of innovation (Coleman, Katz and Menzel, 1966). Second, a more basic question is how the media messages are given meaning by the receivers through their interactions with other individuals. This question is treated in the *convergence communication model* of Rogers and Kincaid, who address the issue not of *diffusion* but of the *creation* and sharing of mutual understanding of information (1981).

Interpersonal discussions are certainly influential, but their influence on HIV/AIDS-related behaviour may increase or decrease the risk of becoming infected. From the prevention standpoint we have to explore the conditions under which networks help or prevent people having accurate perceptions of and reactions to risks.

Norms about Safe Sex

Norms and Sanctions

The information transmitted through social networks pertains not only to events such as sexual behaviour and the occurrence of disease, but also to attitudes and norms. The social network maybe be regarded as the structure that maintains and adapts norms through forms of social control.

What are norms? In a somewhat naive way, they can be understood as explicit, socially standardized prescriptions that actors mention when asked 'what to do and what not to do'. But social reality usually deviates from this ideal pattern. There are important gaps between explicit prescriptions, average behaviour and abstract models. The behaviour of actors is not so much influenced by the explicit norms professed in the subculture as by the perceived behaviour of significant others. In other words, alter's perceived behaviour determines ego's evaluation of the validity or seriousness of norm.

A second question is how this influence operates, how norms arise and how they are maintained. Coleman states, '. . . a norm concerning a specific action exists when the socially defined right to control the action is held not by the actor but by others' (1990). The norm is followed if the actor carries out the action in the way that these controlling others desire. Ego's behaviour, as perceived by others in ego's personal network, may lead to a sanction that is positive when the behaviour conforms to the norm, negative when it is deviant. The degree to which norms are respected depends on the positive and negative sanctions that are applied or expected, and on internalization of the norms. It is important to realize that people seek approval more than they fear punishment. The influence of networks on actors is mediated to a large extent by the fact that approval by 'significant others' is important.

How Do Norms Come to Exist and Be Maintained?

As indicated above, networks can be a means of reinforcing externally produced norms that are transmitted by the media. In the network normative perspective developed here, however, we have to understand how and why norms are created by networks.

Coleman (1990) proposes a rational perspective that tries to explain the conditions under which norms are held by individuals and groups. In such a view, norms give rules for behaviour which are convenient or profitable for the controlling actor(s) or for the group because of the consequences that the behaviour will or is expected to have. A basic assumption in this model is that the consequences of an actor's action are supposed to be collective as well as individual. This basic definition of normative control fits well with contagious disease in general: the behaviour of an individual can affect others as well as the individual. A first step in the elaboration of this perspective is to indicate whose behaviour is interesting to whom. A second step is to understand how norms can be maintained. As Coleman explains, in order for norms to be realized in a social group, the following two collective action problems must be solved: 1) actors must be brought so far that they comply with the norm, even though it is individually irrational for them to do so – each actor would be better off if everybody else complied with the norm, but he alone did as he liked (*the first order of public good*); and 2) actors must be brought so far that they apply sanctions to uphold the norm, even though each actor would be better off if the burden of applying sanctions were borne by all the others without him (*the second order of public good*).

Whether individuals are willing to comply with the norm and sanction others in order to uphold the norm depends to a great extent on their expectations about the consequences of their actions. Whether a person will comply with a norm about safer sex will depend on his or her perception of risks; and a specific cost/benefit assessment of the expected relational sanctions. The pressure to comply with safer sex is stronger when this pressure is exerted in the social field in which the sexual relations are embedded, for example, the social circle of friends.

In this analysis of norms concerning safe sex it is important to identify who is concerned by and thus interested in the sexual behaviour of another individual, and who might be in a position to apply sanctions. As Coleman (1990) stresses, it is not at all automatic for alter to sanction ego's behaviour. Usually, there are costs attached to carrying out a sanction. Alter may find these costs too high and hope that somebody else will perform the sanction. Whether alter applies a sanction when he or she perceives a violation of the norm will depend to a large extent on the costs and benefits to alter of ego's norm violation and of alter's sanction. Different roles as possible sanctioners of unsafe sexual behaviour are played by steady sexual partners, potential sexual partners, and friends or acquaintances who are not viewed by ego as potential partners, as we shall describe below.

Sanctioners as Actual and Potential Sexual Partners

Sexual partners have a special role as holders of norms. For his or her own health, for the quietness and trust of the sexual exchange with ego, alter is interested in ego's behaviour. Alter may find it in his or her interest that ego have no sexual relations at all with third persons. If ego does have sexual relations with third persons, overtly or covertly, then clearly it is in alter's interest that ego's behaviour is *safe*. This implies that alter's problem is to know and control the modalities of ego's relations with third persons. For his or her own interest he or she has first to obtain reliable information on ego's behaviour. In an open sexual market it is problematic to obtain such information. Second, if necessary, alter may try to change ego's behaviour by sanctions, such as showing disapproval, refusing unprotected sexual intercourse with ego, and, finally, refusing ego any kind of sex. These sanctions, however, may be costly in terms of foregoing sexual pleasure and jeopardizing alter's relationship with ego.

If reliable information on ego's relations with third persons cannot be obtained, and/or if alter does not want to incur the possible personal cost of sanctions against a potential love and/or sex partner, then alter's interest needs the intervention of another person. A possible way to obtain such intervention is for alter to try to promote some kind of safe sexual conduct in his or her social milieu. This implies that alter is interested in the general existence and maintenance of a network norm of safe sexual conduct. If such a norm is followed, than alter does not have to bear the risks of sanctioning his or her sexual partner.

There also exists a weaker form of this norm of safer sexual conduct. If ego is part of a social network of persons who are not infected and all these persons' sexual relations are either within this healthy network or (for relations with outsiders) involve safer sexual behaviour, then ego's health is not endangered by sexual contacts. Such a system implies a collective gatekeeping job, i.e., seeing to it that the network remains endogamous or, less strictly, seeing to it that if members of the network have sex with non-members, they protect themselves.

Alters Who Are Close Friends

For alters who are close friends but not potential sex partners, their interest is to have those uninfected with HIV remain uninfected. How can they control these friends? Two forms of sanction are possible. A direct negative sanction is showing disapproval. Indulgence is a value often attached to friendship, and it is often thought that friends should not condemn each other, but friends may have the feeling that, in these cases, criticism means help and solidarity rather than rejection. Furthermore, the sensitive nature of an issue such as sexuality implies that when alter sanctions by exhibiting disapproval this can be perceived by ego as meddling in his or her private life. On the other hand, friends often are the rare persons allowed to be informed of such personal matters. So the values in question are ambiguous, and sanctioning can be costly to alter. A second, but weaker, kind of sanction is more diffuse. Alter could simply tell ego's other friends, acquaintances, or potential sex partners that he or she disagrees with ego's sex life. This is not a very nice but in some cases a quite rational reputational sanction. However, it creates a contradiction, for trust and fairness are basic components of friendship.

Weak Ties and Control

Potential sexual partners and close friends are interested in the behaviour and the health of ego, but sanctioning ego directly is costly for them. The existence of a network norm may permit the escape from the contradiction that the sanctioning endangers the very relationship for the security of which the sanctions would be applied. However, it is difficult to solve the 'second order public-good problem' necessary for maintaining the norm: for whom are the advantages of sanctioning large enough to overcome their costs?

The costs may be lower when the control operates through weak ties in the network. The above-mentioned gatekeeper's job in particular seems possible for social friendship relations who have weaker ties to the ego. Such individuals can try to prevent sexual relations of acquaintances outside the safe endogamous network. Information on sexual relations themselves (who sleeps with whom) is transmitted with less difficulty in the network than information about the precautions taken, so it is less difficult to reduce the frequency of sexual relations with others outside the safe network than to control the safety of such relations once they are there. The weakness of the tie does not decrease the importance of the sanction, because the sanction may be mainly reputational (the controller might speak to others in the network). For the controller the cost is low because the tie is weak. For the controller the advantage may be important; others may be grateful to him, first, for having given information important for their own interest, second, for having imposed a sanction which could have been of very high cost to themselves.

Information and Norms on Sexual Behaviour in Social Networks

As we have seen, information is a particularly problematic aspect of maintaining norms about safe sexual conduct. Information is necessary if a sanction on unsafe sexual activities is to be applied. In addition, information about what is going on will be helpful for the sanctioner to get support from third persons and thus decrease the costs of sanctioning.

In the domain of emotional and sexual matters we have to address a preliminary set of basic question, to wit: Which aspects of an individual's sexual behaviour are known to certain members of his or her intimate or wider social environment? How truthful is this knowledge? And how fast, and with which distortions, is this knowledge further transmitted through the social network? Close relationships and common leisure activities allow members of the personal network of an individual to know the kind of sexual partners exhibited socially by this individual – but no more. Other sexual partners can be hidden from the day-to-day network of acquaintances. At the other end of the spectrum, sexual exploits and, sometimes, sexual practices, are in many subcultures a domain of boasting and window-dressing. From the point of view of prevention, the hidden sexual activities, which are outside the reach of direct social control, are particularly important; while on the other hand overt bragging about sexual activities may have a detrimental effect on perceptions, expectations and norms.

People can talk and disclose to specific others some dimensions of their private lives. A methodological test has shown that people agree to describe with whom, and in what kind of relations, they discuss sexual and emotional matters and how they themselves perceive the sexual behaviour of these confidants (Ferrand, 1991; Ferrand and Mounier, 1993). The answers to such questions in the French national survey on sexual behaviours (Spira, Bajos and ACSF Group, 1993) indicate that 53 per cent of men and 69 per cent of women have at least one person with whom they talk about love and sex affairs. Confidants are mainly friends (same age 37 per cent, different 24 per cent), kin (24 per cent), colleagues (14 per cent). Compared with other data on sociability (Heran, 1988) this shows that not all alters nor all kinds of relation are equally able or allowed to transmit such information.

Norms about the transmission of information about sexual practices can be quite different in different social contexts or social circles. First, norms can compel actors to exchange more or less information which is more or less truthful regarding the kinds of social and sexual lives they have. The availability of information depends largely on how free people are in talking about sex. As a consequence, we can predict that norms on safe sex will be stronger in contexts and subcultures with freedom in talking about sex than in subcultures with a taboo on frank talk about sex, provided, of course, that the perceived risks of HIV infection are not negligible. This prediction means that promoting a free atmosphere to talk about sex and sexual experiences in general, without a necessary reference to HIV or other sexually transmitted diseases, must be an important ingredient of HIV/AIDS prevention campaigns. At the opposite end of the continuum, people involved in married or otherwise steady sexual relationships are often in a context where there exist norms prohibiting any promiscuity or extra-marital sex or any explicit discussion about sex. In such a context there is no established move for applying social pressure, even if accidents occur. Second, social control and possible pressure exerted by the network or portions thereof depend upon the roles that alters can have with respect to ego. The available information, the costs of sanctioning, as well as the effects of the sanctions on ego, depend on these roles. The role and the kind of social context in which a given aspect of ego's sexual conduct is known can facilitate or prohibit intervention by alter in his or her personal or sexual affairs. For example, co-workers can act as if they knew nothing, when friends feel legitimized to say something, and members of the family feel compelled to give explicit advice. So, advice as well as control by the network depends upon the kind of relation between the person and the potential advisor or controller.

Network Structure and Information Flow

As sanctioning presupposes information about ego's sexual behaviour, ego may find it in his or her best interest not to give certain information. He or she can try to manage the information that is transmitted through the network in such a way that approval is maximal and negative sanctions are minimized. However, this management presupposes certain structural properties of the network which depend upon general features of the community.

The more differentiated and the more segmented a community, the more actors can meet culturally and normatively diverse persons, but also the more they can manage their relations in such a way that their networks are non-overlapping. In such a situation, actors can play different roles, and/or it is possible that their (sexual) relations come under the control and approval of only one part of their network. Diverse or even contradictory behaviours are allowed for the same actors if they separate their lives through various circles and special networks, each able to be informed of and to recognize only one aspect of their personal diversity.

Overlapping of sexual networks and the networks of personal friends and acquaintances is more likely to provide greater social pressure. If sexual and non-sexual relations are to some extent mixed in the same network, members can feel more concerned by others' love relationships. For example, networks of friends – where potential sexual partners are often met – are, in many cases, deeply concerned about the sexual lives of the member individuals. In such networks, a norm of free talk can exist more easily. Overlapping also mechanically facilitates the circulation of information. As we have seen previously, it allows diverse actors to share the burden of sanctioning.

Until now, most people who found sexual partners in their day-to-day network of friends behaved as if there were no risk because their day-to-day contacts implied knowledge and trust in non-sexual affairs. This kind of situation and behaviour may be considered dangerous. On the other hand, we can expect that it is also in such structural overlapping of acquaintance and sexual networks that norms of safe sex have a higher chance of being collectively upheld.

Communication and the Emergence of Norms

It is clear to everybody that risk perception is important for norms about safer sex. This has a paradoxical consequence (which is generally present in many questions about the existence of a norm that serves to protect a social group from risks from within the group), to wit, the norm can be maintained only if it is perceived as not being maintained perfectly. If none of ego's potential sex partners is supposed to have risky sexual contacts, then not only is it superfluous for ego to comply with the norm, but it is also superfluous for ego to exert him or her self to maintain the norm. (If ego cares not only for his or her own health but also for the health of his or her friends, then the condition extends also to his or her friends' potential sex partners.) In other words, precisely the networks with the more generalized sexual exchange (the more sexually liberal and, at the beginning of the epidemic, the more risky ones) are more interested in maintaining strict norms of safe sexual conduct and reciprocal control. This means also that it can be predicted that as soon as information about one case of an infected person in a network of potential sexual 'clean' partners begins to spread, stricter norms will emerge.

In social networks that include individuals who engage in sexual relations that are not strictly endogamous, general information about the AIDS epidemic, and more certainly specific information on particular cases of infection will lead to changes in norms about sexual behaviour. The eventual pressure in such a social network towards changes in norms must be great, because unsafe sexual behaviour by other persons, even by persons who may be completely unknown to ego, increases the perceived probability that ego will be infected by HIV. This hypothesis does not suggest that an individual's sexual behaviour is directly affected by the fact of knowing someone infected by HIV. It says only that collective normative pressure will increase with the number of people in the network of friends and sex partners who are informed about significant cases of HIV-infected persons. It is for fundamental ethical reasons that public campaigns urge people not to reject seropositive persons. Nevertheless, it is also possible to suggest that as seropositive people are approached in a more open and friendly way, communication about sexual behaviour and risk will also be more open and norms of safe sexual behaviour will be more strongly supported.

Conclusion

This chapter approaches social life and sexual life not as different domains which interact but as two dimensions of the same reality, i.e., networks of interpersonal relations. Networks are constrained by broader community contexts and they constrain individuals' relational strategies. Four major functions are fulfilled by networks. They

1 relay and personalize public campaign messages;
2 provide a market of potential sexual partners;
3 channel information about personal lifes;
4 produce and support collective norms.

The approach presented here does not treat norms as a kind of exogenous independent variable that can be taken as given, and of which the power and influence on the individual level must be studied. Collective norms are not prescribed by medical or public health agencies, but maintained by groups and networks, on the basis of some collective interest (in the past or present) in their application.

In love relations, because love is love, sexual partners are obviously interested in their sexual partners, others, as alters, in a more detached and cool appreciation of what is going on, are also interested by the health of friends or former and future mates.

AIDS prevention is recognized as a public issue because this disease endangers the population. On the other hand, one's sex life is seen as a private issue. The way in which the question is often addressed creates a conflict between the duty of the state and the freedom of the individual. The basic idea that emerges from the model presented here is that an intermediate level – networks – exists. Because of networks of friends and acquaintances, the behaviour of lovers can be something which interests people around them. A first conclusion is that we have to mind not only how lovers engage in their private relations, but also how people around them are, in fact, concerned by that relationship and can pressure them to adopt safe behaviour.

From this perspective the authors tried to point out some properties of networks which facilitate or impede the emergence of collective norms of safe sexual conduct. The model suggests that the overlapping of friendship and sexual networks is important, but this overlap often appears spontaneously in social life. Another theoretical result can be summarized in a brief sentence: to prevent the spread of HIV, information about personal life must spread through interpersonal networks. A second conclusion, therefore, is that it is important to recommend frank talks as well as French letters.

References

BLAU, P.M. and SCHWARTZ, J.E. (1984) *Crosscutting Social Circles*, Orlando, FL: Academic Press.

COLEMAN, J.S. (1990) *Foundations of Social Theory*, Chicago, IL: University of Chicago Press.

COLEMAN, J.S., KATZ, E. and MENZEL, H. (1966) *Medical Innovation: A Diffusion Study*, New York: Bobbs-Merril.

FERRAND, A. (1991) 'La confidence: des relations au réseau', *Sociétés Contemporaines*, **5**, pp. 7–20.

FERRAND, A. and MOUNIER, L. (1993) 'Paroles sociales et influences normatives', in SPIRA, A., BAJOS, N. et le groupe ACSF, *Les Comportements sexuels en France*, Chapter 6, Paris: La Documentation Française, pp. 171–9.

FISCHER, H. (1982) *To Dwell among Friends: Personal Networks in Town and City*, Chicago, IL: University of Chicago Press.

GANS, H. (1962) 'Urbanism and suburbanism as a way of life: A re-evaluation of definitions', in ROSE, A.M. (Ed.) *Human Behaviour and Social Process*, London: Routledge and Kegan Paul.

HERAN, F. (1988) 'La sociabilité, une pratique culturelle', *Economie et statistique*, **216**, pp. 3–22.

KATZ, E. and LAZARSFELD, P. (1955) *Personal Influence*, New York: Free Press.

MORRIS, M. (1993) 'Epidemiology and social networks: Modeling structured diffusion', *Sociological Methods and Research*, **22**, pp. 99–126.

PETO, D., REMY, J., VAN CAMPENHOUDT, L. and HUBERT, M. (1992) *Sida: l'amour face à la peur*, Paris: L'Harmattan.

ROGERS, E.M. and KINCAID, D.L. (1981) *Communication Networks: Toward a New Paradigm for Research*, New York: The Free Press.

SPIRA, A., BAJOS, N. et le groupe ACSF (1993) *Les Comportements sexuels en France*, Paris: La Documentation Française.

Chapter 2

Norms of Communication and Communication as a Norm in the Intimate Social System

Heinrich W. Ahlemeyer[1] *and Dominique Ludwig*[2]

Introduction

Both in the immediate social experience and in the scientific study of human sexuality, sexual lust and its constraint by norms have formed an almost inseparable unity. The strict social taboos and sanction-amoured norms once associated inseparably with the topic of sexuality (Freud, 1930; Kinsey, 1948), however, have generally given way to less rigid perspectives. In the instrumentalization of erotic lust under the imperatives of achievement and consumption, however, these are often no less alienating than their repressive predecessors (Marcuse, 1970; Nitzschke, 1974; Münz, 1985). ,

The study of sexual behaviour by the empirical social sciences has always had shown immediate connections to the prevailing sexual norms – both in its selection of topics and in its results. The implicit point of reference of quantitative research which dealt with the rates of incidence and the frequencies of particular practices of sexual behaviour – figures which in themselves were without any meaning – was the culturally moulded expectation of normality. Kinsey's famous results of 1948 which showed that more than 10 per cent of the men questioned had experienced homosexual contacts were perceived as a shock because of their contrast to the prevailing sexual norm.

It is the difference between sexual reality and sexual norm which has constituted the leading research interest of quantitative empirical studies of human sexuality (Clement, 1990). This interest has regularly increased at times when sexual norms changed more obviously and rapidly.

The overall liberalization of sexual norms had two important preconditions in society: the general availability of reliable contraceptive devices which diminished, if not eliminated, the risks of an unwanted pregnancy, and the successful suppression of venereal diseases and other health-related risks of sexual intercourse.

If for the brief period of not even twenty years sexuality seemed to have lost its threatening sting and be tamed as a harmless sphere for private pleasure and pure enjoyment, the appearance of the HIV and the discovery of the epidemiology of AIDS has reunited what for a short period could appear to be two completely distinct spheres of life: *l'amour et la mort*, sexuality and death.

AIDS is a sexually transmitted virus infection which ultimately leads to death. In spite of slow progress in the care and therapy of AIDS patients, the disease cannot be cured once an organism is infected with the HIV. As long as a systematic vaccination against the virus is not available, primary prevention is the only effective way of breaking the dynamics of the spread of the HIV. As heterosexual transmission accounts for nearly 60 per cent of actual AIDS cases on a global scale, the policy of prevention has to aim at modifying particular patterns of sexual behaviour that have been identified as the main channels for transmitting the virus, such as unprotected vaginal and anal intercourse (Enquetekommission, 1988).

If sexual behaviour and its social constraint by norms have long been treated almost as a unity (Schelsky, 1955; Christensen, 1971), the question arises whether HIV prevention efforts could use normative means in order to bring about the desired change in sexual behaviour. We want to discuss the significance and limitations of the norm concept for understanding the actual process of intimate communication in general and preventive behaviour in particular. The leading question that gives orientation to our reflections asks about the contribution of the norm concept to improving practical preventive efforts against the spread of HIV among the heterosexual population.

The scientific cooperation over borders of discipline and theory needs common reference points. Such a reference point could be found in each other's research material: transcripts of in-depth interviews with men and women about their sexual encounters which in spite of differences in focus, method and language displayed immediate parallels and complementations. An excerpt from an interview with a German woman typically reflects – as both contributors agree – the problems of communication and interaction in intimate situations. This example will lead to an outline of the different theoretical orientations of the contributors: the system-oriented sociological approach and the social psychological approach. The article is concluded by the major results of the discussion between the authors specifying where they see convergences and differences of their approaches in dealing with the norm issue.

'... and I trust you too'

An unmarried twenty-seven-year-old woman from a medium-sized German university town falls romantically in love with a (German) man she has met three months ago during her vacation on Korfu, Greece. After exchanging glances and a smile the first night at the bar, they 'happen' to meet again at the bar the next night, start talking to each other and decide to have dinner together in a 'southernly romantic realm'. They go to her appartment afterwards 'not in the intention of sleeping together, and yet it happened'. On the advice of her girlfriend, she had bought condoms for the first time in her life and took them with her, but she does not use them:

I: 'I think this happens to many people at that moment . . . you don't think of it. It's really too bad.'

Q: 'You said you talked, in fact, about AIDS before sleeping together. Can you remember what you actually said?'

I: 'Yes. When it became obvious to me that we were going to make love, I brought the conversation round to condoms, which I had packed into my suitcase, but with him there was such an aversion, perhaps because, I don't know whether one may say it that way, no matter who brings up this subject, the other one will take it as a motion of no-confidence, like: I want to protect myself, I don't know what is the matter with you. I don't know how I would react if someone said to me: not without condoms. Then I would say: you think I got AIDS or what?'

Q: 'Did your friend react like this?'

I: 'No, no, but I would have reacted that way. No, he did not react that way. He asked why I had them at all, and I said, well, if something was gonna happen and such, and . . . yes, because of the whole AIDS thing and such, yes. But he didn't go into it at all. He essentially just said: "You know I didn't sleep with anyone for some time and I trust you too".'

Q: '. . . and with that it was clear to you that the condom remained in the suitcase or how did it go on?'

I: 'Yes, also because of the handling; I know little of it; and anyway, even though I never tried them, I always imagine that to me it is an interruption' (ISYS interview #18/p.14).

I: 'We talked . . . so that both of us felt: we can trust each other, and it is this trust which made the way open for us to make love with each other. Not necessarily that . . . sure, we talked about AIDS, that you could feel secure and only then I will sleep with you, and such . . . that wasn't even it. Also that I had condoms with me and such, that one was really just . . . yes, at that moment it was: look, I'm a modern woman (laughs). On my side, it was not at all meant seriously, not really; just: I am following and, rubbish, I shouldn't have brought them in' (ISYS interview #18/p.17).

The System-oriented Sociological Approach

In the intimate interaction shown in the interview transcript above, a number of prerequisites for successful AIDS prevention – as discussed in the literature

– are given: (1) *information*: the respondent is well-informed about AIDS and its possible risks; and (2) perceives it as personally relevant to herself (*concern*). (3) As a consequence, she wants to act in a preventive manner (*intention*). (4) She does not rely upon good intentions only, but actually gets active and buys condoms. She quite correctly supposes that condoms are an appropriate means of HIV prevention and that it may be important to have them handy (*availability*). (5) She even manages to make AIDS and the use of condoms a subject of the conversation with her new partner before the intimate encounter (*communication*). And yet, despite five prerequisites of successful AIDS prevention being fulfilled on the side of the young woman, ultimately preventive action does not take place, if the use of condoms in sexual encounters is defined as the decisive indicator of a successful AIDS prevention.

The interview excerpt above is paradigmatic of the conspicuous discrepancy between a high level of knowledge about AIDS, about its transmission, protective methods and widespread preventive intentions on the one hand and a widely practised non-preventive sexual behaviour on the other. To put it more sloppily: AIDS has obviously changed a lot in the heads, but little in the beds.

This difference between theory and praxis, intention and factual behaviour is to a large extent attributable to the effects of the mutual interaction of partners in the course of the intimate encounter, that is to say: to the social dimension of intimate communication. As Pollak (1991) pointed out, individual-centred concepts, as the health belief model (HBM), have brought some light into particular components of dealing with AIDS-related risks, but: 'being centered on the individual, the HBM neglects the dynamic social interactions that shape behaviour' (1991, p. 74). With the absence of a direct relationship between an individual's level of knowledge and attitude towards AIDS and behaviour, further research on sexual behaviour and the risks of HIV infection 'clearly requires *focusing on the specific social interactions that influence individual behaviour*' (Pollak and Moatti, 1990, p. 25).

The determinants for AIDS-related behaviour changes can be identified not just on the level of the individual, its attitudes and knowledge, and on a macro-societal level, but also on the intermediate level of the mutual interaction of intimate partners (Luhmann, 1982). To grasp the particular social dimension of sexual behaviour and AIDS prevention, the research at the ISYS takes up the present state of sociological system theory (cf. Luhmann, 1984) and conceptualizes the interactive dynamics between two intimate partners as a *social system of intimate communication*. It is on this level where a common preventive modification of behaviour either succeeds or fails (Ahlemeyer, 1990).

To describe sexual behaviour as a social system implies its analytical decomposition. It becomes possible to take up recent findings on social systems in general and specify them for the particular field of sexual behaviour.[3] One basic discovery about social systems refers, for instance, to their elementary mode of operation: as closed systems, they organize their reproduction according to self-produced internal states and structures. In contrast to former assumptions of an immediate determination of systems by the environment, this concept emphasizes their autonomy and internal self-organization.

In order to enter into a relationship with their environment, social systems first have to take care of their own continuation from moment to moment. So it is only on the internal basis of their elementary operations that they can develop a relationship with the environment (Luhmann, 1984). This concept has far-reaching consequences for every attempt of a preventive intervention from outside: it emphasizes the difficulties of prevention which in its effects depends on an autonomous process of understanding on the side of the intervened system. It is the intervened system which defines the conditions under which it admits to become impressed from outside. Preventive interventions can only be successful with regard of and consideration for the autonomy of the intervened system (Willke, 1987).

Searching for ways of improving strategies of primary prevention of AIDS, means that it becomes a prerequisite to gain an understanding of the autonomy of sexual communication systems and analyse more closely what is perceived as useful information. So what constitutes the closure, the basic mode of operation of intimate systems? How do they consequently observe their environment? How do AIDS-related risks appear on the internal monitors of the system? And which preventive consequences can be observed in actual behaviour? These are the four main questions that the research project at Münster seeks to answer.

In contrast to other social systems such as neighbourhood or working relations, the distinctive unity of intimate systems lies in their orientation to sexual interactions of the participants so that their communicative design is out for an integration of the physical-sexual dimension. Intimate systems are systems (1) which as self-organizing communicative systems dissociate themselves from their environment; (2) which are oriented at integrating a physical-sexual environment; and (3) therefore have to engage in constructing an erotic reality in contrast to the everyday reality (Davis, 1983).

Beyond this unity and particularity which characterize intimate systems in contrast to non-intimate systems, there are four different types of intimate communication systems which have evolved today: (R) romantic; (H) hedonistic; (M) matrimonial; and (P) prostitutive systems. These four types of intimate systems differ fundamentally (1) in the systemic closure of their elementary operation mode (autopoiesis); (2) in their form of self-organization and their internal structures; (3) in their observation of and relation to their environments; and (4) in their observation of AIDS-related risks and the possibilities and difficulties of participants to put preventive options into practice. These four types of intimate communication, which claim to cover the totality of heterosexual intimacy, thus predefine different conditions for improving preventive efforts against AIDS.

All HIV-relevant heterosexual interactions take place in either of these four intimate systems.[4] Rape as a social pathological variant of H, M and P is, however, to be treated separately. Intimate social systems do not consist of real 'persons', but of communicative elements which are selectively reproduced. The intimate system can be imagined to extract from the participants those actions necessary for the ongoing reproduction of the system from moment to moment or, equally, to omit those which might endanger or cease a continued system operation.

Not rarely, it occurs that one and the same person participates, with different actions, in different intimate systems. A married man has sexual relations with another woman and occasionally visits a brothel. According to the requirements of the intimate system in question, this person behaves differently towards AIDS-related risks according to whether he is in the marriage bed, in the bed of the mistress or in that of a prostitute. In a system-oriented research, the objects are thus not individual persons or actions, but the differential structure and patterns of intimate communication systems which form individual behaviour.

The ultimate elements of intimate systems are communications which are attributed as acts to participating persons. The ultimate elements are highly temporalized events which vanish in the moment of their constitution. Temporalized elements from the very beginning are out for something else to follow. They can only actualize in event-like combinations and therefore from moment to moment create new situations. The main concern of such a system built as a network of fleeting self-produced events has to be securing the 'connectivity' of its elementary operations, shall it not simply cease to exist – a case which is not so rare with love relations or marriages.

Intimate dyades are thus *autopoietic systems* which constantly produce and reproduce their elements of which they exist. Systems of this kind are immanently restless; they are exposed to a dynamic that is endogenously produced. An adequate point of reference for analysing them is thus not balances or other static states, but the continuing reproduction of momentary events the systems consist of.

Which act follows upon another one cannot be left to coincidence or arbitrariness alone. No system could manage an entropic state of complete indetermination of one moment to the next one. This applies even more to intimate systems which consist of events, of vanishing elements, and which have a very large amount of possibilities at their disposal and thus display a high structural complexity. In all cases, the system will develop *structures* in order to limit what can follow upon what. By specifying structures, the system individualizes itself. Everything which helps to bridge the gap between one event and the next acquires the function of a structure in the system. The structure of social systems generally consists of *expectations*. The prostitute is available for money; by their own initiative, men do not make a move to touch contraception as a topic. Expectations emerge by limiting the scope of possibilities and even permit to include their own disappointment.

Expectations produce the alternative of becoming either true or disappointed. Dealing with disappointment, there are two general ways of handling expectations: a normative and a cognitive mode. Expectations ready for learning are *cognitions*. One is ready to change them if reality turns out to be different and unexpected: the girlfriend has her period. Expectations unwilling to learn are *norms*. In the case of their disappointment, they are upheld against the facts: the wife has a lover, and yet she is expected to be faithful. The normative mode of expectation produces the difference of conforming and deviant behaviour.

Norms pose requirements of participation in clearing the situation: a readiness to reinstall the norm at least in the form of explanations, apologies or lies. Sanctions and explanations are institutions of handling disappointments; their function is to renormalize the situation after it has occurred (Luhmann, 1984, pp. 437–56).

The concept of intimate social systems thus does not take vantage from normative presuppositions, but introduces norms on a secondary level. Its prime concern lies with the continuing autopoiesis of the system from moment to moment by its own operations. Norms are of interest to the extent that they give structure to the self-reproduction. This abstinence in regard to a norm-centred concept does not mean that social life in general and sexual relations in particular were possible without norms. The self-commitment to norms and values is, it is true, a pervasive act of social life, particularly in a sphere where expectations are as risky and susceptible to disappointment as in sexuality.

At the same time, however, norms do not just 'exist' as such: they are produced and reproduced as part of the communication system to which they are specific. If norms are but a special case of structures by help of which a system reproduces itself from one moment to another, empirically a distinction has to be made between four different sets of communicative norms which are specific to the social context in which they occur: the norms of romantic, of hedonistic, of matrimonial and of prostitutional intimate systems. Norms of agents outside the intimate system have a communicative relevance only to the extent that they are constituted within the system. This also applies to norms entrenched into the psychic systems of the participants involved.

The Cognitive Social Psychology Approach

In cognitive social psychology, research focuses upon the individual's internal thought processes and thoughts. Since the development of the cognitive theoretical perspective within psychology, the *responding* subject of the behaviourists has been conceptualized as an active builder of the world in which he perceives, thinks, feels and acts. According to cognitive psychologists, individuals are conceived as reacting to psychological realities they create, rather than some objective independent stimuli. For instance, a partner's characteristics could be considered by a behaviourist as a cause of preventive responses, whereas the determinant for a cognitive social psychologist would be the subject's perception of the partner's characteristics.

In cognitive social psychology, this theoretical revolution initiated the extended scientific study of the individual's internal thought and perception processes. Within social psychology an impressive field of research developed, known as the *naive, intuitive, everyday* psychology. Together with advances made in artificial intelligence, the field developed some basic laws of reasoning, such as the use of routine mental operation, shortcuts, heuristics and the categorization of new information in pre-existing schemas, with the attendant risk of distortion. In this perspective, real thinking occurs on those few occasions where new information fails to fit pre-existing categories. Perceptions often do not take into account all available information. They sometimes do not even consider the pertinent information. If totally consistent decisions were the goal, the everyday thinker makes many mistakes. This pessimistic view seems inevitable because the cognitive orientation focuses more on the internal processes and results than on the social situations where the processes and results are produced (Forgas, 1981).

In spite of disappointment about cognitive orientation and the pessimistic view of man as a poor thinker that seems inevitable when mostly isolated individuals are studied and rules of functioning are compared with norms of science (Beauvois and Croyle, 1984), some advances from social cognitive psychology are to be kept in mind. The great characteristic about processes involved in perceiving and thinking is the human being's extraordinary ability to organize and process information quickly, thus allowing rapid behavioural adaptations. This seems to be especially true when social interaction processes are considered. As Heider observed in the 1950s, people are especially good at social behaviour, 'The complexity of feelings and actions that can be understood at a glance is surprisingly great . . . "Intuitive" knowledge may be remarkably penetrating and can go a long way towards the understanding of human behaviour' (1958). Scientists have much to learn from ordinary people in matters of sex and love, where people are all but naive.

Although AIDS-related psychosocial research is highly concerned with information processing, man cannot be considered only as a thinker, neither in his aspirations nor in his functioning. Other components of conduct, besides cognition, must be taken into account, and the literature is full of controversies because different theories make different assumptions about whether knowing, feeling, evaluating, or acting best predicts behaviour (De Montmollin, 1984). Some of these theories question the predominant implicit notion that human action is guided mainly by reason. Our own research perspective is that the affective, evaluative, connotative and behavioural components may be considered different levels embodied in real conduct. Each of these components can become determinant of the others, depending on the circumstance, and none must be eliminated in order to shed light on the richness of potential conducts.

Recently a renewed interest in affect has become perceptible (Cooper and Croyle, 1984), but the affective part is not often considered in the predictive models that are available for health prevention research, and desire is still completely omitted. Even if one is convinced of the value of such theoretical models as the theories of planned behaviour, reasoned action and Health Belief Models (Rosenstock, 1974; Taylor, 1986), when explaining individual behaviour under volitional control, it is still uncertain whether they can be applied in predicting HIV-related behaviour, where strong affective determinants, such as sexual desire and love, obviously play an important role (Pollak and Moatti, 1990). Moreover, some important questions are left open. For instance, if risk perception is considered a determinant of preventive behaviour in HBM, how is risk perception itself to be explained?

Social psychology's main contribution to preventing the further spread of HIV may be the study of understanding. First, a lack of understanding of the public discourse on HIV and AIDS could prevent people even being interested in prevention, or, if they are interested, comprehending preventive information correctly and agreeing with preventive recommendations. Second, understanding intervenes in actual expressed interactions including those required by direct protective behaviours.

Improvement of preventive public discourse relies upon systematic knowledge of what people have in mind about AIDS. What notions of HIV risk are used by ordinary people? What contents are common? Which are unexpected? With what criteria do individuals explain why at this time they used condoms, but not at other times? To answer these questions, qualitative research has to be done from the point of view of the actors rather than the epidemiologist. The concept of the individual as anticipating, imagining and creating fantasies and rehearsing before acting (Gagnon, 1988) is very important when inquiring how people get prepared to participate in sexual encounters and engage in preventive actions.

Ordinary people in their own context use their common sense, a kind of *sufficient* knowledge, different from an expert definition of a *better knowledge* based on science. All social cognitive theories insist upon the fact that this common sense is made of organized stockpiles of knowledge, which guide action and interpersonal relations. What types of knowledge should then be taken into account when studying HIV risk reduction? What are the components of a situation upon which everyday understanding relies? What do people bring into their interactions with their partners? How do situations come to make sense?

These questions confront the psychologist with the concept of meaning rather than thinking. When individuals' perceptions of situations are accorded careful attention in the qualitative analysis of empirical data (Ludwig, 1990; 1994), the focus is first on knowledge other than that directly related to HIV transmission and prevention, for instance, knowledge related to factors of good health, to other sexual risks such as pregnancy, being seduced, isolated or loved. Such factors might be considered inappropriate from the epidemiological point of view. However, they are hypothesized to be critical in helping people adjust to their lives, in which AIDS is not necessarily of critical importance.

That is why our own research focuses first, more on intra-individual rather than on inter-individual differences; focuses more on *when* than *who* questions. Second, when we examine realities as they are experienced by subjects, the roles of contexts and situations are emphasized. This leads us to ask how individuals make sense of specific situations. For instance, what is meant by telling a sexual partner, 'I am thinking about AIDS' or 'I want to have safe sex'? In determining meaning, cultural norms add some meaning to the situation that is beyond the immediate consideration of isolated individuals.

According to social representation theory (Moscovici, 1961), symbolic and real social exchanges produce shared realities, which in turn facilitate communications. Their roots in collective memory give social representations an historical and a cultural dimension. For instance, the ambiguous social object AIDS might be linked with previous well known notions such as *epidemic* and *syphilis* (Jodelet, 1989). In this way it becomes more familiar, while at the same time assuming different meanings for different social groups.

Since culture often adds meaning without our being consciously informed of it, the study of historical and anthropological dimensions is important. True, this is outside the psychosocial domain, but norms, defined as prescriptive standards and acquired through socialization, are among the most significant aspects of culture (Krebs and Miller, 1985). In Lewin's group dynamics they have been defined as a field force and have been suggested to be an important component in promoting individual behaviour change.

Since norms and related concepts frequently appear in the empirical data that is collected about sexual risks (Memon, 1990; Siegel and Gibson, 1988; Spencer, 1984), they are hypothesized to be an important part of common-sense knowledge about specific situations, often associated with affective repercussions, belonging to the training of the social actors, and providing resources for coping. Among different normative concepts are the influence of behavioural standards or rules which are more or less prescriptive and sanctioned. In addition, there is a wide range of other ways norms intervene. For instance, the belief that peers are not using condoms may inhibit some potential preventive efforts when sexual partners belong to the same social group. Even cognitive expectations may have normative effects in intimate communication. New concepts such as *schema* describe what is commonly expected, and that of *script* describes the expected temporal sequences of events. Labelling a sexual encounter as normal or abnormal has consequences on several aspects of conduct such as risk perception and emotional states.

At the individual level, only a special configuration of multiple factors is likely to explain protective behaviour (Ludwig, 1993). The concept of interaction, which is related to the concept of social influence, occupies a central place in social psychology. The discrepancy between knowledge and behaviour in almost all studies about AIDS that we have reviewed (Ludwig and Touzard, 1990) can be explained partly by the neglected interaction processes that transform what is expected to occur from individualistic characteristics and internal processes. We constantly and unconsciously adapt to others. I react to what I think you think, to what I think you are, to what I perceive from you, etc. In return, you react to my reaction, and subsequently I react to your reaction, and so on. Yet this is only a very simple translation of what occurs in a real interaction. Thus the sexual situation is hypothesized to be permanently defined in the interaction between partners.

Social norms intervene in these specific interactions in several ways. Social norms and values are present in language, thus in negotiations dealing with prevention. Norms are also related to social influence. As is shown in experimental studies about social influence, norms and values can affect the type of consensus resulting from group discussions (Moscovici and Doise, 1992). Normative beliefs may affect sexual partners' efforts to deal with prevention. The influence of others is acknowledged to be crucial in acquiring healthy behaviour such as quitting smoking or drinking. This influence of others has been proven to increase with uncertainty, as is the case with AIDS.

Different types of social influence, in which norms play an important role, may be applied to the study of specific interactions dealing with HIV prevention. In one situation, the norm of 'real' love, implying a total giving of self, may help convince a partner to have unprotected sex, even if he or she wanted to use a condom. In another situation the norm 'in the time of AIDS everyone shares the responsibility of protecting health' might exist. This norm would be more supportive of protective behaviour.

While sexual interaction is one of the most strongly socially regulated areas of human behaviour, it also belongs to the most private sphere, in which partners are allowed to set their own norms. In sexual relations a sort of consensus or compromise has to be found, especially if protective behaviour is to be adopted. Of the various ways to negotiate with others, Sherif's normalization process (1969) may be applied to a range of situations in which external objective criteria are missing. In this case, a common point of reference results from the reciprocal interpersonal influence. This could fit intimate communications to the extent that partners have equal status.

The study of norms and values appears to be crucial in understanding individual and relational aspects of HIV-risk behaviour and, thus, conceptually necessary to improve prevention. However, for both theoretical and methodological reasons, this objective is difficult to achieve. Since correlations do not necessarily indicate a causal relationship, except in cases of observable transgressions of the norm, a particular conduct cannot easily be inferred to be caused by social norms. When studying the influence of norms, one must differentiate their relative importance according to the temporal sequence and the type of relationship under consideration. Internalized rules of behaviour and normative expectancies seem to be more effective in the beginning of a relationship, when the self-image is confronted with a somewhat unknown and desired stranger. Particular norms are then drawn up jointly afterwards, as a specific relationship is established. The more important the relation is to the individual, the more he or she becomes sensitive to the image conveyed to the other person.

Discussion: Convergences and Differences

We decided to sum up the major results of our exchange on concepts, methodology and empirical cases under the aspect of convergences and differences. The two approaches were seen to converge in the following points:

1   *Scope and comprehensiveness of approaches*
    The common object of our respective analyses is heterosexual intimate encounters with a special focus on the issue when preventive behaviour succeeds and when it fails. If the use of condoms looks at first glance like a simple yes or no question, it is all but trivial both in a social psychological and a sociological perspective. Condom use in intimate encounters turns out to be a result of a multiplicity of social and psychological factors and their particular configuration in the situation. Neither of us claims to offer a comprehensive model answering all the questions involved. However, the concepts presented set out not only to suggest new answers to the well-known issues of prevention, but also pose these questions in a new manner.

2   *The observability of norms*
    Norms – both in a psychological and a sociological sense[5] – pose to their scientific description particular problems which have to do with their very nature. If norms are, as sociological systems theory suggests, expectations upheld after their disappointment, their normative mode often becomes apparent only with their transgression or violation. As complicated rules of behaviour – the taboo of talking about AIDS or condoms, for instance – they hardly become empirically apparent as long as they are observed. Innumerable situations touch on normative expectations without displaying their normative imperative. It is just 'normal' that people are dressed. It is only when a norm is violated that its content and impact become manifest: you must not run around nakedly. Norms are often weaved so intricately into the texture of language and into what is taken as 'normal' that they are hard to detect – both for the social actor and the scientific observer.

3   *Empirical observations*
    Analysing each other's research material showed that on a descriptive level there are a number of striking parallels and similarities in the course and structure of intimate encounters – in spite of given differences in research design, focus and methodology. Three examples illustrate this:

a) Rarely are there examples in the research material where a man and a woman who have not known each other before have sexual intercourse immediately the first time they meet. Some familiarity between partners seems to be a prerequisite, and it is gained not only by communication (see point 6), but also by the use of additional time which is integrated between a first and second encounter.

b) It is to the woman to propose preventive action: both in the French and the German sample a marked 'inequality' in the 'division of labour' between the sexes is striking. Even when both men and women acknowledge the necessity of preventive action, it is nearly always the woman who raises the issue of contraception or AIDS and who opens the way for the use of condoms. Men are not only more hesitant in addressing these problems, but also attempt to avoid the use of condoms once they have been mentioned. This holds true for all kinds of different intimate systems.

c) If condoms are accepted and used in the very beginning, of a heterosexual relationship, both in the German and the French sample a strong tendency can be observed to leave the condom out afterwards. With increasing familiarity, the risks of an HIV infection begin to disappear for the partners so that after a few meetings they no longer find precautionary measures necessary any more and leave them out altogether. Only in a small minority of cases is this step preceded by a common AIDS test which takes the time for sero-conversion into account.

4   *The fragility of intimate systems*

Intimate social interaction demands the creation of an 'erotic reality' which is distinguished from the ordinary activities in everyday life. Only to the extent that the wide-awake world of work, plans and figures, of duties and sorrows is faded out does it become possible to generate and stabilize an erotic reality with its own meanings, symbols and dynamics (Davis, 1983).

Everyday reality and erotic reality constitute two distinct realms which have little in common and tend to exclude each other. The unexpected appearance of components of the erotic realm in everyday life often creates disturbances, annoyance, embarrassment or even shocks. Intimate communication, on the other hand, is highly vulnerable to the impact of everyday reality. Minor signals may suffice to make the sexual intercourse collapse or prevent it from getting started: the ringing of a telephone, the news on the radio, a creaking bed, pending problems of everyday reality, the mention of contraception or AIDS.

Intimate systems continue only as long as they are able to constitute and keep up a difference to everyday reality. As everyday reality tends to force itself in many ways on lovers, intimate systems are highly fragile – threatened by collapse and destruction through a different reality at almost any moment. A highly focused attention and active contributions to the common construction of an erotic realm is thus demanded of the participants. This often implies attempts at avoiding components that have been experienced as particularly destructive to the erotic realm in previous encounters.

5 *Communication as a norm*

The complexity and multiplicity of factors involved in sexual interaction comprises three basic levels: the organic, the psychic and the social. Each level plays a distinctive indispensable role. In the empirical material collected, the organic encounter of bodies in the sexual act between a man and a woman who did not know each other before is always prepared on a social level by verbal communication. Depending on the stage of progression, however, non-verbal communication acts, such as glances, smiles, airs or posture, play an equally important role.

In order to gain at least a minimum of familiarity, the partners 'have to talk' – about the disco, the weather, themselves, their musical preferences, whatever. The act of talking with each other prepares the psychic systems involved in the physical encounter of the bodies and renders it acceptable. A quotation of the account of a female respondent of the German survey may illustrate this point:

'I was expecting visitors, and he had holidays and had come to see me, and *we had got so marvellously into talking* – which surprised him in a way because he is usually rather reserved, and then he said: "I'll stay until your visitors arrive," and then they came, and the whole time, *we had talked so wonderfully. It was a smashing conversation.* And when it rang, I got up and wanted to answer the door. And somehow it came over me. I took his head into my hands and kissed him on his mouth, very affectionately . . . And when I came back to him – and this I found just super; I think I am still being amazed by it – he took me in his arm, embraced me and kissed me so sweetly' (#16, 40/41).

It is only by the intensive communication between the partners that the way for a first sexual encounter becomes viable.

6 *The communicative preparation of condom use*

The use of condoms is not simply a technical act, but it bears immediate consequences for various aspects of the sexual act. Most of all, it requires a communicative preparation of the partners. Even where condom use has become an obligatory part of a professional routine, as with prostitutes working in brothels, there is usually a short explanatory sentence about it before the act: 'You lie down there and relax, and I will put this on to you.'

As it is not possible to conceal the use of condoms from the partner, it usually takes at least a short verbal agreement or even negotiation about the integration of the preventive device into the situation. Without having talked about it at all, it is very difficult to bring the condom in. If it is introduced without any communicative preparation, disturbances and embarrassments have to be expected at a later stage.

The ability to talk about the condom with a new partner is eased by preceding talks about it with friends or parents. There are individual aspects, for instance experience and self-confidence, as is indicated by a high proportion of self-reliant men and women over thirty-five who have little difficulty in addressing the subject. And there are systemic aspects, as it takes the investment of confidence in the other person to expect the acceptance of the proposal. As the excerpt from interview #18 above illustrates, this confidence is at the same time discouraged by the idea that the other one might take the proposal as a 'motion of no-confidence'.

7 *Symbolic meanings of the condom*

Whether or not the condom is perceived as a viable alternative that can be introduced into the intimate situation is also contingent on the perception and interpretation of the condom. If it is perceived as a symbol of '*le rapport sexuel*', of pure sexuality, it is hardly acceptable for those who seek an effective commitment of 'love'. If it is perceived as a reminder of the existence of AIDS and death, it has little appeal for those who seek fun, excitement and life. If it is seen as a 'selfish' protective device against the other one, it offers little encouragement for those who are striving for community, trust and confidence. If it is seen as something that keeps two people physically and sensually separated, it has little attraction for those who want a total fusion. If the condom is seen as a symbol of everyday reality, its chances are small to be introduced into a reality that is experienced as clearly distinct.

There are, on the other hand, connotations and contexts which ease the use of condoms. If introduced for the purpose of contraception, they are much more acceptable than for the purposes of AIDS prevention. The thought of pregnancy, even an unwanted one, seems to fit in more easily with intimacy than the mention of AIDS, which evokes images of disease, suffering and death.

The proposal of condom use is also eased if brought in with the argument of protecting the partner: 'I suggest we use a condom in order to protect you.' In this form, it is a motion which can expect a greater chance of acceptance with its reference to altruism as a generally appreciated norm. This proposal, however, may not be available to men and women alike. While it is acceptable for a man to display having had several female partners before, this is generally not yet the case for women.

8   *Temporal structures*

Time plays an important role in the sexual act. Problems of prevention are, for instance, not the same before or after the sexual act nor are they alike in the beginning of a new relationship or later. Both samples show numerous cases where the partners talked easily about contraception and HIV afterwards but did not address the issues when it would have made sense from the point of view of the health system.

As to the three different systems involved in the sexual act – the organic, the psychic and the social level – the hypothesis is proposed that while each level is involved in every moment of the encounter, there are different phases in which each system assumes a predominant role. In the beginning, the psychic system of the participant seems crucial in a preceding decision whether or not to seek or accept an approach to a potential partner. After this has been decided in the positive, the social system takes over. It is by communication that the partners get to know each other and prepare the sexual encounter. In the sexual act, finally, the actions and reactions of the organic level gain an autonomy of their own kind and determine what happens. Verbal communication occurs in this stage only as a means of increasing sexual arousal or as a 'repair mechanism' for treating problems which have occurred on the organic or the psychic level.

9   *The rationality of intimacy and the rationality of the health system*

From the point of view of the health system, it is well justified to regard the use of condoms as the most effective form of HIV management. As a precaution that reliably interrupts the transmission of the virus from one body to the other, it may be seen to be more effective than strategies to reduce the number of situations to exposure, as promises of strict faithfulness or intentions of practising sexual abstinence (Pollak and Moatti, 1990, p. 26).

Empirically, a wide scope of different behaviours towards the risks of the HIV can be found ranging from just thinking of it and doing nothing in the situation on one end of the scale to the consequent use of condoms on the other. Between these two extremes, there are many other forms of what is seen as precautionary behaviour: speaking of the risks of AIDS – often with the adverse effect that talking about it has created so much community and familiarity that it no longer seems necessary to actually take AIDS-preventive measures; the selection of a particular partner by avoiding persons from major risk-groups or attempts to investigate the past of the partner; a reduction in the number of intimate partners; intentions or promises of strict monogamy; problem solutions in a chronological dimension, such as the installation of additional time in order to get to know the new partner more closely before having sex with him or her; undergoing an HIV test, alone or together, with or without regard of the intermediary time for a sero-conversion; demanding that the partner submit to a test or produces a certificate with negative test results; a modification of sexual practices by the avoidance of particularly risky behaviour, as penetration during menstruation periods, anal intercourse or a complete abstention from penetration.

Which behaviour is actually chosen is to a large degree a reflection of the particular 'rationality' of the intimate relationship. This rationality may differ profoundly from the scientific rationality of the health system. In the perspective of the intimate system, AIDS-preventive behaviour is but one question out of a whole range of issues which confronts the couple. In view of the fragility of the intimate system, the constant threat of collapse posed by everyday reality and its dependence on achievements of other system levels, such as the organic and the psychic, it may be perfectly 'rational' not to propose and use condoms in the intimate situation with a new partner, whereas in the perspective of the health system such a behaviour may look careless and irresponsible.

The rationality of the health system comprises a long-term perspective and is able to refer to accepted values as scientific truth, reason and health. It is easily congruent with the general notion of rationality, with which the demands of the intimate system, on the other hand, seem to be incompatible. And yet it is important to note that the concern with erotic lust and pleasure, immediate experience and concentration on the very moment are representations of a rationality of its own kind. From the point of view of the scientific observer of both the health system and intimate systems, neither of the two rationalities may be described as 'superior' in the sense that it could substitute the other one. They have different reference points and serve different functions.

In discussing our concepts and data, we identified particular problems in which we saw our approaches diverge. The following issues could not be resolved and are proposed for further elaboration:

1   *Two different norm concepts*
    The common use of the term 'norm' in sociology and in social psychology tends to conceal the distinctive meaning of the norm concept in each of the scientific disciplines.

    As a social psychological notion, it refers to evaluated preferences which operate in psychic systems of individuals in imperatives like 'you should . . .' or 'you must not'. The focus lies with the internal mental processes of the individual and the respective role of cognitions, representations and what is held as 'normal'.

    In a system-oriented sociological approach, norms are a particular form of the structure of social systems: expectations which are upheld even after their disappointment. Here, the point of reference is not the socialized individual and its internal processes, but the ongoing operation of communicative systems. The sociological norm concept thus binds both the existence and function of norms to their communicative constitution which implies normative representations by language, signs and symbols.

Neither do the two different norm concepts claim a right of exclusive representation, nor are they incompatible. They do have different analytical focuses which throw light on different strata: the psychic and the social reality.

Systems-oriented sociology demands a normative abstinence of the researcher in the sense that research must not follow predetermined 'normative concepts', but rather observe the social forms in which sexuality takes place and find out the particular function and significance of social norms.

2 *Different perspectives*

Among the most interesting parts of our common work were the discussions of empirical cases and data in which the differing perspectives of our disciplines became apparent.

Social psychology deals more with what the individual brings into the situation and what content and processes he shares with others as a member of his group and culture. It thus focuses on shared processes and contents of individuals which they bring into the situation.

System-oriented sociology deals with the social level that is constituted by the emergence and continuing operation of communicative systems. Their elements are not individuals or men, but communications which are attributed to individuals as (communicative) actions.

As a consequence of the two differing disciplinary approaches, there is a difference in focus. Whereas the sociologist's interest is aroused with the emergence of the intimate system, the social psychologist's interest starts with preceding perceptions and decisions of the individual. S/he asks, for instance, how individuals categorize situations according to the dimensions of 'love' or 'sex' and how this categorization interferes with risk perception in specific encounters.

As different as these two disciplinary perspectives may be, they allow particular achievements and are complementary rather than irreconcilable: social psychology can complement the social system perspective, for instance, by the concept of 'the rehearsed individual'; and sociological systems research can open new perspectives radically different from those of the individual.

3 *The significance of norms*

In correspondence with our different theoretical and methodical vantage points, we come to different conclusions about the significance of norms in shaping sexual behaviour and, consequently, in improving AIDS preventive strategies.

For social psychology, norms have many significances. One of their most important functions is to offer a point of reference by help of which evaluations and judgements are made. Individual judgements and evaluations are made about social relations which are compared to this point of reference. Whether or not these relations are in congruence with normative reference points is not only of relevance for determining the type of communication between intimate partners, but also for the actualization of behaviours.

For the sociological systems theory, social norms are but a particular mode of dealing with expectations by which social systems gain structure. In intimate relations, their main function is to help to solve system problems of continuity, warding off the constant threat of collapse which is posed by everyday reality. In their ubiquity, they are hardly discernible and often become apparent only after the disappointment of expectations. Outside norms are of social relevance to the extent that they are communicatively represented within the system.

It is one of the particularities of sexual norms that their very transgression may be discovered to constitute a vital source of lust and pleasure, a very component of eros itself (Dannecker, 1987).

Whereas these reflections tend to limit the significance of norms for social systems in general and intimate social systems in particular, they assume, however, an important function in AIDS-preventive policies. The preventive messages have to observe and be compatible with the norms of the intimate relationship addressed, if they are to get a chance of being heard, considered and transformed in intimate interaction. The relative success of AIDS prevention in gay communities would have been impossible without an unreserved acceptance of the norms and values of homosexual men, most importantly homosexuality itself (Peyton, 1990). This experience may be immediately relevant for addressing the participants of heterosexual relations outside the legitimate social forms of romantic love and marriage, such as prostitutive and hedonistic relationships.

It is one of the contributions of system-oriented sociological research on sexuality to keep in mind that even if these communicative prerequisites of prevention are given, their realization remains ultimately dependent on autonomous operations of the intimate system whose decisions may be stimulated, but not determined by the health system from outside (Ahlemeyer, 1993).

This stimulation is strongly aided by a close observation of what actually happens in intimate relations and in the psychic systems involved. The research conducted both in Münster and Paris has produced extensive material on this which has not yet been analysed with reference to the issues outlined in this chapter.

Notes

1 The research on intimate social systems conducted at ISYS – Institute for Systemic Social Research at Münster – is funded by a special grant of the BMFT Research Promotion of the AIDS-Zentrum des Bundesgesundheitsamtes Berlin (FK V-007-90). Heinrich W. Ahlemeyer is obliged to the members of the research team at ISYS and to Wichard Puls and Dirk Richter in particular for their helpful comments on earlier drafts of the manuscript.
2 Dominique Ludwig worked at the Laboratoire de Psychologie Sociale of Université René Descartes, Paris, she died in 1994.
3 The elementary operation of social systems is communication. We speak of communication whenever a distinction is made between information and notificative behaviour. Simple perception allows for a high degree of a simultaneous distinctions. Communication, on the other hand, requires a considerable dissimultaneization from perception. The resulting sequence of information processing in communication results in the construction of a new complexity: the constitution of social systems.
4 The concept presented here only refers to heterosexual behaviour. While the topology seems to be of some use in order to understand the interactive dynamics of homosexual couples too, this needs further reflection and elaboration, especially because of different sets of meanings in homosexual and heterosexual social contexts.
5 Cf. the discussion of two different norm concepts.

References

AHLEMEYER, H.W. (1990) 'Intime Kommunikation and präventives Handeln: Über einige soziale Voraussetzungen der Primärprävention von AIDS', in ROSENBROCK, ROLF and SALMEN, A. (Eds) *AIDS-Prävention*, Berlin: Sigma, pp. 181–8.
AHLEMEYER, H.W. (1993) 'Aidsprävention als Systemintervention: Konturen des Zusammenhangs von intimer Kommunikation und HIV-Risiko-Management', in LANGE, C. (Ed.) *AIDS–Eine Forschungsbilanz*, Berlin: Sigma, pp. 197–210.
AJZEN, I. (1988) *Attitudes, Personality and Behaviour*, Buckingham: Open University Press.
BEAUVOIS, J. and CROYLE, R.T. (1984) *La Psychologie quotidienne*, Paris: PUF Fondamental.
CHRISTENSEN, H.T. (1971) *Sexualverhalten und Moral*, Hamburg: Rowohlt.
CLEMENT, U. (1990) 'Empirische Studien zu hetereosexuellem Verhalten', *Zeitschrift für Sexualforschung*, **3**, pp. 289–319.
COOPER, J. and CROYLE, R.T. (1984) 'Attitudes and attitude change', *Annual Review of Psychology*, **35**, pp. 395–426.

Heinrich W. Ahlemeyer and Dominique Ludwig

DANNECKER, M. (1987) 'Die Lust am Verbot', in *Das Drama der Sexualität*, Frankfurt: Athenäum.

DAVIS, MURRAY, S. (1983) *Intimate Relations*, New York: Free Press.

DE MONTMOLLIN, G. (1984) 'Le changement d'attitudes', in *Psychologie Sociale sous la direction de S. Moscovici*, Paris: PUF Fondamental.

ENQUETEKOMMISSION (1988) *AIDS: Fakten und Konsequenzen. Endbericht der Enquete-Kommission des 11. Deutschen Bundestages*, Bonn: Bundestag.

FORGAS, J.P. (1981) 'What is social about social cognition', in FORGAS, J.P. (Ed.) *Social Cognition Perspectives on Everyday Understanding*, European Monographs in Social Psychology Series, New York: Academic Press, pp. 1–20.

FREUD, S. (1930) 'Das Unbehagen in der Kultur', in *Werke*, Frankfurt/Main: Fischer, Bd. IX, pp. 191–270.

GAGNON, J.H. (1988) 'Sex research and sexual conduct in the era of AIDS', *Journal of Acquired Immune Deficiency Syndromes*, 1, pp. 593–601.

GAGNON, J.H. (1989) 'Disease and desire', in *Daedalus*, 118, pp. 47–77.

GERHARDS, J. and SCHMIDT, B. (1992) *Intime Kommunikation. Eine empirische Studie über Wege der Annäherung und Hindernisse für 'safer sex'*, Baden-Baden: Nomos.

HEIDER, F. (1958) *The Psychology of Interpersonal Relations*, New York: Wiley.

HUBERT, M. (Ed.) (1990) *Sexual Behaviour and Risks of HIV Infection*, Brussels: Publications des Facultés universitaires Saint-Louis.

HUBERT, M. and VAN CAMPENHOUDT, L. (1990) 'Perception du risque de transmission sexuelle du VIH, modifications des comportements et contexte sociale et familial', in JOB SPIRA, N., SPENCER, B., MOATTI, J.P. and BOUVET, E. (Eds) *Santé publique et maladies á transmission sexuelle, des voies de recerce pour l'avenir*, Colloque INSERM, Chamonix: John Libbey Eurotext, pp. 183–9.

JODELET, D. (1989) *Les représentations sociales*, Paris: PUF Fondamental.

KAPLAN, H.B., JOHNSON, R.J., BAILEY, L.A. and SIMON, W. (1987) 'The sociological study of AIDS: A critical review of the literature and suggested research agenda', *Journal of Health and Social Behavior*, 281, June, pp. 140–7.

KINSEY, A.C., POMEROY, WARDELL B. and MARTIN, CLYDE, E. (1948) *Sexual Behavior in the Human Male*, Philadelphia: Saunders.

KREBS, D.L. and MILLER, D.T. (1985) 'Altruism and aggression', Chap. 14 in LINDZEY, G. and ARONSON, E. (Eds) *The Handbook of Social Psychology*, 3rd edn, New York: Random House.

LUDWIG, D. (1990) 'Analyse de quelques réactions au SIDA dans une population étudiante', in JOB SPIRA, N., SPENCER, B., MOATTI, J.P. and BOUVET, E. (Eds) *Santé publique et maladies á transmission sexuelle, des voies de recerce pour l'avenir*, Colloque INSERM, Chamonix: John Libbey Eurotext, pp. 512–15.

LUDWIG, D. and TOUZARD, H. (1990) 'Sida, transitions individuelles, Revue de question', *Revue Internationale de Psychologie Sociale*, 3, 1, pp. 127–39.

LUHMANN, N. (1982) *Liebe als Passion*, Frankfurt: Suhrkamp.

LUHMANN, N. (1984) *Soziale Systeme. Grundriß einer allgemeinen Theorie*, Frankfurt: Suhrkamp.

MARCUSE, L. (1970) *Triebstruktur und Gesellschaft*, Frankfurt: Suhrkamp.

MEMON, A. (1990) 'Young people's knowledge, beliefs and attitudes about HIV/ AIDS: a review of research', *Health Education Research*, **5**, 3, pp. 327–35.

MOSCOVICI, S. (1961) *La psychanalyse, son image et son public*, Paris: PUF Fondamental.

MOSCOVICI, S. and DOISE, W. (1992) *Dissenssions et consensus: Une théorie générale des décisions collectives*, Paris: PUF Fondamental.

MÜNZ, R. (1985) 'Sexualität in Beziehungen. Eine Rekonstruktion auf Grund biographischer Interviews mit österreichischen Frauen', in HUSSLEIN, HUGO, OLECHOWSKI, RICHARD and RETT, ANDREAS, *Sexualität als Entwicklungsproblem*, Wien: Herold, pp. 118–82.

NITZSCHKE, B. (1974) *Die Zerstörung der Sinnlichkeit*, München: Kindler.

PEYTON, J. (1990) 'Bedingungen und Verlauf der AIDS-Aufklärung für schwule Männer in San Francisco', in ROSENBROCK and SALMEN (1990) pp. 321–6.

POLLAK, M. (1988) *Les homosexuels et le SIDA. Sociologie d'une épidémie*, Paris: A.-M. Métaillié.

POLLAK, M. (1991) *AIDS prevention for men having sex with men: Final Report*, Lausanne: Institut universitaire de médicine sociale et préventive.

POLLAK, M. and MOATTI, J.P. (1990) 'HIV risk perception and determinants of sexual behaviour', in HUBERT, M. (Ed.) (1990) pp. 17–45.

ROSENBROCK, R. and SALMEN, A. (Eds) (1990) *AIDS-Prävention*, Berlin: Sigma.

ROSENSTOCK, I.M. (1974) 'The health belief model and health preventive behavior', *Health Education Monographs*, **2**, pp. 354–86.

SCHELSKY, H. (1955) *Soziologie der Sexualität. Über die Beziehungen zwischen Geschlecht, Moral und Gesellschaft*, Hamburg: Rowohlt.

SHERIF, M., SHERIF, C.W. and HOLTZAN, N.G. (1969) *Social Psychology*, New York: Harper and Row.

SIEGEL, K. and GIBSON, W.C. (1988) 'Barriers to the modification of sexual behavior among heterosexuals at risk for AIDS', *New York State Journal of Medicine*, February, pp. 66–70.

SPENCER, B. (1984) 'Young men: Their attitudes towards sexuality and birth control. Family planning and society, *British Journal of Family Planning*, **10**, pp. 13–19.

TAYLOR, S.E. (1986) *Health Psychology*, New York: Random House.

WILLKE, H. (1987) 'Strategien der Intervention in autonome Systeme', in BAECKER, D., MARKOWITZ, J. and LUHMANN, N. *Theorie als Passion: Niklas Luhmann zum 60*, Frankfurt: Suhrkamp, pp. 333–61.

Chapter 3

Relationships between Sexual Partners and Ways of Adapting to the Risk of AIDS: Landmarks for a Relationship-oriented Conceptual Framework

Benoît Bastard, Laura Cardia-Vonèche, Danièle Peto and Luc Van Campenhoudt

Introduction

The object of a good deal of social science research on AIDS is to assess the way in which individuals handle the risk of being infected during sexual relationships. What motivates two partners to enter into a relationship? What factors come into play to favour or prevent them from addressing the possible risk of HIV? How do partners behave when they ultimately take action and have sexual intercourse? What attitudes lead partners to use or stop using means of protection that have been proven medically reliable? What circumstances lead partners to believe that they do not constitute a threat to each other? These questions will be addressed in this text using as a base two qualitative studies, one done in France and Switzerland and one in Belgium. Our objective is theoretical, that is to suggest an outline for modelling some of the key factors that must be considered to understand how partners handle the risk of AIDS in their sexual relationships.

When we refer to 'the way of coping with the risk' or 'the way of adapting to the risk' we are talking about the whole array of perceptions partners form and the types of behaviour they adopt with respect to the problem of AIDS in relationships they establish. These ways of coping thus cover different aspects of communication about the risk and the concrete methods of protection practised, such as use of condoms or the HIV screening test, as well as rationalization processes and language justifying and accompanying these practices. As for communication, we consider the question of whether partners have addressed the issue together, and in what way: before or after the first time they have intercourse; in a general and evasive manner (mentioning the spread of the epidemic and its risks for society and other people); or in a precise and detailed way; concerning their own situation, etc. With regard to practices we consider whether the risk is managed or denied.

In the first case we consider how condoms are used: Are they used systematically or not? Right from the first time of intercourse or later on? For how long? Are they abandoned after a few times? We also examine how tests are used: Does one consider that being tested is a prerequisite to sexual relationships, or is it seen as a means of reassuring oneself after the fact? The second case brings us back to the question of the justification of behaviour in which risk management is lacking.

We are interested in the whole set of factors, including the rationalization processes and language used in prevention, that help shape people's perceptions of the epidemic, how it is spread and appropriate means of protection. These perceptions can lead to relativization of the risk based on the idea that the disease presents no danger for partners depending on their social background or sexual habits, the type of relationships they get involved in, or means of spreading attributed to the epidemic. Or they may lead to an approach to the risk, reinforced by beliefs about how the disease is spread, and, for example, by the fact that it strikes people 'we know directly' (Von Allmen, Bastard and Cardia-Vonèche, 1993).

Different ways of adapting to the risk, such as communication, practices, and justification, are all connected. For example, our work suggests that there is a greater likelihood of engaging in preventive risk management when individuals address the issue of AIDS when they enter the relationship than when they start to have sexual intercourse without communicating with each other on the subject. One may also think that the total lack of concern in sexual relationships is often linked to a line of argument that downplays the risk of AIDS. For example, some individuals feel the risk of infection is being amplified by the media, and is, in reality, much smaller than other risks, such as the risk of a traffic accidents or the risks inherent in atomic power plants. Hence, one of our aims is highlighting some of the factors enabling us to explain ways of coping with the risk of HIV infection and their various facets. When do we see a tendency to raise the problem and possibly take preventive measures? When is there a search for *relational safety*, due to partners' belief that the routes of the disease's transmission as they see them and/or the circumstances of their relationship rule out any possible danger? Finally, when do we observe a total lack of concern for the risk of AIDS?

We can start to conceptualize these questions through the discussion of five factors:

1 the type of respective partner's involvement in the relationship;
2 the stage of the relationship and partners' positions in their life cycles;
3 the social space of the relationship;
4 the balance of power in the relationship; and
5 the relationship with one's body and perceptions of health in relationships with others.

Benoît Bastard, Laura Cardia-Vonèche, Danièle Peto and Luc Van Campenhoudt

The choice of factors was based on the assumptions that risk-related behaviour depends, first, on the characteristics and dynamics of the relationship between partners, and, second, on the relationship partners have with their bodies and with their health.[1]

For the first and fifth factors we shall base our findings on the French-Swiss research, and for the other three factors on the Belgian study. In both instances the research was qualitative, based on semi-directed discussions with 40 or 50 men and women involved in heterosexual relationships. Consequently, the findings remain largely exploratory due to the samples. The Belgian research included men and women from 19 to 60 years of age who had changed partners recently or had several partners at the time. The French-Swiss sample included only men and women who had already lived with someone but were living alone at the time of the survey after recently ending a relationship.

The way the five factors are presented and studied depends on the epistemological and theoretical perspectives of the research teams. The French-Swiss team wanted to establish and verify a direct relationship between how partners commit themselves to their relationship and how they see their bodies, on the one hand, and the ways they cope with risk, on the other hand. The Belgian team builds a typology of ways of coping with risk that enables a better understanding of what goes on in certain problematic situations, such as the young man's anxiety in his difficult exploration; the feeling of security produced by separating worlds; responses to the crisis; and the risk run by the dominated woman (Peto *et al.*, 1992). This work does not aim to establish cause-and-effect relationships between explanatory factors and behaviour. Factors, such as the stage of the relationship, the social area of the relationship or the balance of power between partners represent critical aspects of the relationship for understanding the sexual behaviour related to HIV risk. These factors contribute to understanding why it is normal behaviour from the partner's perspective.

Given these differences in the teams' approaches, we do not construct a unified explanatory model. Rather the two teams bring some of their respective findings together with a view to making progress in conceptualizing partner-interaction related to HIV risk behaviour.

The Factors

Types of Involvement in a Relationship

How individuals dedicate themselves to their relationships is the first set of factors we consider. This is the *relating to others* dimension. We feel that the type of commitment to a relationship is crucial for understanding the manner in which partners communicate about AIDS, and we test this in two ways.

First, we differentiate relationships according to the level of expectations partners have of them. An essential factor might be the desirability of the relationship, which may vary with fluctuations in the size of the market of potential sexual partners. We hypothesize that some people who are in a committed relationship would like to discuss AIDS with their partners or use condoms but are hampered from doing so because they fear such requests might be taken the wrong way, and call the relationship into question. Conversely, others who are not strongly committed to the relationship (since they have alternatives) might have less difficulty bringing up the issue of AIDS, as they would not be afraid of harming the relationship.

Second, we might look at a relationship's expectations from the standpoint of content rather than their intensity. Indeed, these expectations take on meaning in a more general way of relating to others. We have suggested a method of characterizing these patterns based on the current trend of analysing family interactions and exchange in the couple (Kellerhals and Montandon, 1991; Troutot and Montandon, 1988; Von Allmen, Bastard and Cardia-Vonèche, 1989). We characterize the ties binding two partners by making the distinction between individuals living in *fusion* or *associative* relationships. A fusion relationship highlights togetherness and is based on the durability of a relationship. It puts emphasis on the assimilation and the interdependence of individuals and adhering to family values and beliefs such as fidelity and mutual commitment. Fusion relationships are notably characterized by the idea of total sharing in all areas of life. In contrast, associative relationships are characterized by individuals who define the areas of exchange in a relationship and how this exchange is to be implemented. Partners negotiate the terms of the contract binding them. Not all aspects of daily life, for example, social life or leisure activities, are necessarily encompassed in this exchange. Emphasis, thus, is on differentiation and the independence of the individuals within the couple.

Distinguishing between these types of couples hypothetically enables us to grasp more clearly the ways in which individuals communicate with each other about AIDS. In fusion relationships the romantic dimension is predominant. We hypothesize that this makes any questions about the other partner's relationships with others and preventive practices difficult. For associative relationships, on the contrary, we hypothesize that there is an inclination toward a system of transparent exchanges whereby it is possible to share past experiences and discuss the risks taken in the relationship.

We note that there are two different levels to these conceptualizations. The first is the macrosociological perspective, which makes the rarity of potential partners on the market a barrier to expressing concerns about prevention. The second is more slanted toward the microsociology of the couple's functioning and considers the fusion mode to be an obstacle to prevention, whereas the associative mode is hypothesized to allow for the expression of concerns about health.

Our hypotheses were not confirmed by our data. We observe that some partners show an attitude of consideration of the risk and others do not, regardless of how tight the market may be and whether the relationship is fusion or associative. For example, young people, who, by definition, are on a very open market with a possibility of extending the network of relationships to a great many partners, do not usually take precautions suggested to reduce the risk of HIV infection. We tested the second model's validity using the data from the French-Swiss team (Bastard and Cardia-Vonèche, 1992). Fewer than half of those involved in an associative relationship actually brought up the question of AIDS at the beginning of the relationship, or so they say, whereas more than half of those in a fusion-type relationship brought up the subject. The negotiating space in an associative relationship is not necessarily used for discussing sexuality or AIDS, whereas partners in a fusion relationship may unveil secrets and transparency which may bring them to talk about every problem, even the risk of AIDS.

While our hypotheses have not received empirical support, we do not want to dismiss too hastily the idea of the 'relating to others' dimension as a way of understanding the means of coping with risk. The problems may be methodological. How might we have conceptualized the risk more relevantly? Are there particular contexts in which associative or fusion relationships would predict risk-related behaviour?

Stage of the Relationship and Partners' Positions in their Life Cycles

In the broad sense, a sexual relationship is not limited strictly to intercourse. It also includes all aspects of communication and interaction between partners that precede and surround sex, allow sex to occur and give it structure. The relationship is presented as a dynamic process that is transformed and recomposed in time (Goffman, 1974; Huston and Levinger, 1978; Padioleau, 1986). Ways of adapting to the risk of HIV and AIDS may largely depend on the stage of the relationship. According to the Belgian study (Peto, *et al.*, 1992), the stage of the relationship is, in many cases, a crucial factor in determining behaviour patterns. Three relationship phases were identified in the Belgian study: 1) courtship–seduction; 2) familiarity; 3) unravelling phases. Each stage is associated with specific phenomena in the relationship that may present obstacles to the use of condoms in relationships or may result in some risk.

The predominant concerns during the *courtship–seduction phase* are to present the best image, win trust and avoid sources of conflict. These concerns take precedence over that of protecting oneself from the risk of AIDS, which partners may tend to minimize. Many respondents have testified that they understood the risk of certain behaviours in contributing to HIV infection and would like to use a condom, but they abandoned the idea at the slightest sign of reticence from their partners. As a result, situations in which the risk is totally eliminated at the first encounter are in the minority, at least among this study's respondents. The *familiarity phase* corresponds to a situation in which partners have already had sex, feel they know each other and have established ties bringing them closer together. In many cases this is the stage where the relationship is felt to be stabilized, whether it has been going on for several years or only a few days. For several reasons, this impression can also get in the way of risk management, especially the use of condoms. We observe that familiarity is generally associated with safety, there being a tendency to consider those close to us as safe, while strangers are potentially dangerous. Homogamy among partners reinforces this impression. But we particularly note how difficult it is to manage the risk and hence how difficult it is for most people to introduce suspicion into a relationship which requires trust in order to be built. The paradox of this situation is that in some cases the risk of AIDS makes love stronger in the sense that taking risks, far from being avoided, may be sought out, as it is emotionally functional.

In sexual relationships the feeling of familiarity is established extremely quickly compared with other types of relationships, such as professional or neighbourhood relationships. This is due to the 'self-disclosure' (Reiss, 1986a; 1986b) process and the intimacy implied by sexual intercourse and the context, including nudity, closeness of contact, etc. In our work, like other studies, it is common to observe that those who used condoms the very first time most often abandoned them after only a few times. Even during the *unravelling stage*, when partners thought their relationship was coming to an end, we observed that the use of condoms, or of other means of prevention, remained unlikely between partners who were used to having intercourse without taking precautions, unless the decline in their relationship was specifically linked to at least one of the partners having had or having a relationship perceived to be risky.

The stages of a relationship take on different meanings according to the points partners have reached in their life cycles. This factor considers where the individuals are with respect to their personal emotional, sexual and/or marital history, as well as their place in the relationship. This dynamic has been considered by several other investigators (Gagnon and Simon, 1986) as a key factor in behaviour with regard to risk. In the Belgian study, five phases in the life cycle were identified, as follows: 1) discovery–exploration; 2) search-for-lifestyle; 3) stabilization; 4) deconstruction; and 5) celibacy. Each position in the life cycle corresponds to specific psychological moods and roles, particular responsibilities and a set of given constraints. They are in no way connected in any chronological order, except the discovery–exploration phase, which comes before the others and corresponds to the discovery of shared sexuality. Thus, apart from the discovery–exploration phase, individuals may, quite to the contrary, experience myriad transitions from one phase to another in varied sequences throughout their lives.

In this text, where the emphasis is on the relationship rather than the individual, we shall show how the stage of the relationship and position in the life cycle interact according to the situation. We hypothesize that when a relationship is in the courtship–seduction stage and brings together partners who themselves are in the discovery–exploration phase, image and avoiding conflicts become very important. For example, in the case of those initiating a relationship, the fear of making a bad impression and losing the partner's trust takes great precedence over the concern of protection from AIDS. These people will tend to deny risk and make an after-the-fact rationalization to justify their taking this risk and to reassure themselves. For some, selecting a safe partner is based on criteria that is not very effective, such as physical appearance and associations. This phase is also characterized by less social control, due to the absence of a socially recognized partner, such as a spouse or steady companion. There is a greater potential to have several partners without having to answer (too much) to one's peers. Conversely, a man or woman in the stabilization phase is more or less committed on a long-term basis to a stable relationship with a socially recognized partner. Extramarital affairs are usually conducted more or less discreetly and may even carry a feeling of guilt, unless they are accepted by the stable couple, with varying behavioural scenarios with respect to the risk of AIDS. To explain behaviour in these phases we must introduce the notion of the primary or secondary space of the relationship.

Primary or Secondary Space of the Relationship

The distinction between the primary and secondary space allows an examination of the attitudes toward risk in sexual relations by giving an important place to the relationship and, at the same time, accounting for the relationship's context. Each sexual relationship has its own rationality and its own life. However, what goes on in it is not independent of other relationships partners may have. For example, a married person may have one or several other partners he or she sees discreetly. The significance of these relationships, how they are conducted and behaviour in response to the risk of AIDS may not only be very different from one situation to the next (for example, according to the stage of the relationship), they may also vary according to what is happening in the partners' other relationships. To explain these differences and the processes of tension between parallel relationships we use the distinction, made in urban sociology, between primary and secondary space (Remy and Voyé, 1981). The primary space is the *official space* where the individual is influenced by the power of accepted authorities and, to a greater or a lesser degree, to various forms of social control over the fulfilment of work, community, home, school and other roles in society. In contrast, the secondary space provides a background of anonymity away from the ordinary social controls, a *counterspace* where it is possible to step outside instituted roles, to be and do *something else*, perhaps with other partners (downtown, in a foreign country, the private club, a roadside bar, sauna, etc.).

The exploratory work done in Belgium (Peto, *et al.*, 1992) reinforces our idea that the distinction between these two types of space is relevant for explaining relationships between partners and, in particular, the way in which they consider the risk of AIDS. Firstly, the rule of homogamy where 'birds of a feather flock together' is more likely in the primary than the secondary space. The nature of the power struggle between partners is largely contingent on the degree of homogamy; the more heterogamous partners are, the more lopsided their relationship. Consequently, the way in which they react to the risk of AIDS will depend more on partners' respective assets and their abilities to capitalize on them.

The norms of a sexual relationship also vary in terms of the primary or secondary space of the relationship. Generally speaking, trust is the prevailing norm in the primary space due to homogamy between partners. Consequently, suggesting the use of condoms may look like a show of mistrust. In the secondary space, norms of the relationship vary more (since the partner may be a lover or a mistress who means a lot or may be the partner in a one-night stand). On the other hand, norms for the framework of a relationship may be imperative to keep the relationship from being exposed in the primary space. Thus, it is enough for one partner to need to keep the relationship secret for him or her to lay down the law if, by chance, the other partner wants the relationship to be out in the open (for example when one person is married and the partner is single). For the same reason, a married partner may consider using a means of contraception with his or her spouse but may not necessarily choose condoms in an extramarital affair. However, it is not enough to compare what goes on in the primary and secondary space by juxtaposing the two spaces, for what matters most in partners' behaviour with regard to risk is the constant tension between these two poles.

The quest for secondary space may be all the more intense the less complete life is in the primary space. Yet this tension does not necessarily lead to sexual intercourse outside the primary relationship. One might wonder, in fact, whether the sex trade, which provides sexual satisfaction without sexual intercourse (peep shows, videos, magazines, etc.), does not have the function – at least for some people – of completing the primary space without having to face making the efforts and taking the risks inherent in parallel relationships. Moreover, the very nature of sexual practices in the secondary space seems linked to established behaviour patterns in the primary space. Thus, far from being avoided, risk may be systematically sought out in secondary experiences when life in the primary space seems too monotonous and conventional (Levi-Makarius, 1974). Several perfectly socially integrated people replied that they sought out what they judged to be a reasonable dose of risk and challenge in their secondary experiences (Peto, *et al.*, 1992). Thus it appears that the more highly structured the primary relationship, the more difficult the primary–secondary tension, and hence the approach to the inherent risk in secondary relationships, may be to manage.

Balance of Power between Partners

The study of sexual relationships and their effective norms requires the consideration of the balance of power between partners. This notion will be examined briefly based on the notion of capital structures (see Bourdieu, 1972). We feel that the way partners negotiate over their behaviour with regard to the risk of HIV depends on their comparative capital structures. Four types of capital structures are distinguished: *economic*; *social*; *cultural*; and *symbolic*. How are they relevant to the power balance between sexual partners? *Economic* capital can be mobilized directly, for example, to move from the primary space, set up circumstances for a favourable meeting, seduce the partner, make the other person financially dependent, or pay for the latter's services, in which case it is likely to impact behaviour strongly. *Social* capital refers to the network that can be mobilized by individuals to find multiple sexual partners or to exert pressure on each other through friends or significant others. In sexual relationships, cultural capital takes various forms, such as communication skills and social skills. For example, talking with ease about sexuality and AIDS and being comfortable with one's body may be derived from having the necessary social skills. *Cultural* capital has the power to overwhelm the other partner's beliefs. For example, we came across the case of a middle-aged man who was considered by his partner to be cultured. He was very well informed about the risks of AIDS but deliberately underestimated the risk with one of his young ill-informed conquests in order to have intercourse without a condom. Lastly, *symbolic* capital is defined as the capacity to use the types of capital mentioned above to create a strong value in the eyes of the partner. For example the prestige, appeal of money, power, and education and treating oneself to costly cosmetic care can be translated into what we commonly call charm, beauty, sex appeal and, more generally speaking, youth. In emotional and sexual matters symbolic capital can often be exchanged for sex or at least be used in the transaction of sexual intercourse. The use of capital resources have not yet been verified systematically and empirically, nor have they been made operational. They are presented as ideas requiring further study and clarification.

Relationship with the Body and Means of Health Management

The ways in which people get involved in sexual relationships and handle the risk of AIDS are linked to their relationships with their bodies and their approach to health management. This dimension seems to be mobilized when trying to find out how we cope with disease. Boltanski (1968) refers to the relationship with the body as the manner in which we nurse it, develop it, fortify or embellish it through sport and various corporal practices, and are more or less attentive to the unpleasant and unusual sensations it registers. The elements constituting the relationship with the body pertain to its role in one's appearance and seduction in love relationships in particular (Boltanski, 1968; Cardia-Vonèche, Von Allman and Bastard, 1987; Dodier, 1986; Osiek-Parisod, 1990). We shall now discuss the impact of the instrumental and reflective relationships with the body. These two principal types of relationships with the body have been defined and their importance has been shown by Boltanski (1968).

The relationship with the body is said to be instrumental when the body is seen as a tool which enables the individuals to meet their professional and domestic obligations. It usually functions without one's realizing it or taking special care of it. Health in such a relationship with the body, 'is nothing more than a customary state, which merits neither attention nor reflection' (Boltanski, 1968). Health management consists of reconstituting physical and intellectual capacities, meaning the individual reacts only when the body fails to meet expectations, and manifests itself through pain or illness. This is an anomaly, a twist of fate, that must be resolved as quickly as possible and usually leads to interventions that re-establish the habitual course of life. The system is driven by a repair logic. In an instrumental relationship with the body this mechanism leads to the emphasis being put on the ability to attract by conforming to certain expectations of a partner for seduction and taking the appropriate corrective measures when expectations are not met. With respect to sexuality it is when standards are not met that special attention is given to performance as well as breakdowns.

Conversely, in a reflective relationship to the body, individuals consider their bodies as one would an aesthetic object. Hence, the body is seen as something worthy of attention and observation. It becomes an object of constant care, through proper diet, sport, etc., in order to conserve it over time. For people who have this type of relationship with their body, health is a good that can be controlled; being sick is a sign of some defect in one's life-style, of something lacking in prevention practices; respecting the body's rhythm is necessary for taking care of oneself. Seduction is based on maintaining a satisfactory self-image, which is considered to be a necessary precondition for seduction skills.

We hypothesize that these contrasting types of relationships to the body have opposite effects on the way the risk of AIDS is approached and managed. Sexual exchanges are characterized by concern for forethought and prevention for people in the reflective mode, whereas they are characterized by a degree of fatalism and reparative logic for those in the instrumental mode. As in the case of some of the hypotheses about types of involvement in the relationship, these hypotheses were not confirmed by the Franco-Swiss research. While roughly two out of three of the people having a reflective relationship with their body showed attitudes of real concern for the risk (they either used medical means for protecting themselves or explained that they had appraised the partner, weighing the risks that were entailed), we found that an almost identical proportion of people having an instrumental relationship adopted the same attitudes and showed a true awareness of the problem. Some reflective people whom we would have expected to heed prevention messages have adopted very strict attitudes to the risk of AIDS which seem contradictory to the way in which they take care of their health in other areas of their lives. For example, they do not bring up the issue of AIDS in the relationships they form, deny the risk and criticize the importance placed on information about the epidemic. This is quite unlike the people who protect themselves from the risk of AIDS, one way or another, while having an instrumental relationship with the body. What motivates the latter to adopt protective behaviour is the desire to manage their relationships as they see fit. Some indicated, for example, that they used condoms to protect themselves from problems that might arise with their partner, whether it be pregnancy or other health problems. The use of precautionary measures is linked to a concern for keeping a large degree of freedom in the relationship and not feeling committed. A condom is thus used, in a way, to keep the partner at a certain distance. These people do not want anyone meddling in their plans for life, nor do they want to be restrained in their desire to change partners. In practice, they are motivated to adopt protective behaviour by relationship-oriented, not health-related, concerns. What seems to be a preventive attitude isn't, and there is not the stable, constant connection we imagined between the relationship with one's body and the way of handling the risk of AIDS.

The reason that our hypotheses have not been confirmed may be that HIV/AIDS and the risks it presents are not considered problems of prevention in most relationships. Only a small group of individuals conceive of sexual relationships like other aspects of life, in terms of health. The majority do not feel that they are faced with the problem of comparing health concerns with those of getting involved in new relationships. Sexual relationships are merely seen from the angle of the intimacy and pleasure they provide. Paradoxically, the information from this hypothesis essentially strengthens even more our conviction that we need to study further risk-related behaviour based on analyses of relationships, in the true sense of the term, and the ways partners get involved, rather than characteristics peculiar to the subjects, such as the relationship with the body, which might be considered in themselves, separate from the relationship.

Discussion

Concerns about Health and Means of Involvement in Relationships

Following this examination of these five factors, we can discuss how health concerns versus the expectations from relationships influence the ways people adapt to the risk of becoming infected by HIV. We started with the belief that some elements of the relationships posed an obstacle to the introduction of health-predicated behaviour. We assumed that individuals considered health concerns to be something outside the relationship that often presented an inherent conflict of interest with the desire for sexual intercourse. It seems we must break away from this conception if we want to understand better the sexual behaviour of individuals with respect to the risk of HIV infection. We now believe that health concerns and behaviour apparently relevant to prevention are, to a great extent, the expression of relational strategies. However, the aim of handling the risk is not necessarily health preservation but part of the relationship's language. For example, there are different strategic uses for condoms. In some instances it is used for keeping a distance from the partner and showing the limits of the relationship. In other instances it is used to show respect for the other partner's desires and to reassure them. Not using condoms also has a strategic sense. It may be dictated by the concern for safeguarding pleasure or not complicating matters at the beginning of the relationship by a difficult discussion. It may also be the expression of the wish for increased intimacy and total mutual trust. The use of condoms then is a type of information for the partner regarding the state of the relationship.

Communication about an HIV infection and the possible risk it carries is a revealing test of the relationship. The issue of AIDS is encompassed in the array of communication problems facing couples. Each interaction may have many meanings and may be seen as strengthening or, on the contrary, challenging the relationship. Talking about AIDS may be perceived as a sign of trust or, conversely, as the expression of distrust of the other. Not talking about it may be seen as a sign of love or, on the contrary, as a show of irresponsibility. The problem of AIDS is not external to a relationship, but is often one of the relationship's constituents. The different manners of handling the risk that we have brought forward are not stable results of factors pertaining to relational patterns or health, whatever the complexity given to these factors' arrangement. They make up one way of expressing the state of the relationship. Consequently, they may change over time, depending on what becomes of the couple, or vary for the same individual from one relationship to another.

Trying to Give an Explanation – Should we Throw in the Towel?

Given these considerations, is it possible to define a way the respective factors studied above explain HIV risk-related behaviour? Broadly speaking, we believe there is no reason to be hopeful that we can build a comprehensive, predictive model of cause and effect regarding the ways of handling the risk of AIDS. The factors of intelligibility have not yet been sufficiently studied and possibilities for combining them are very complex. Their respective weights vary from one situation to another, so that a central factor in a given situation, like the position in the life cycle, may appear totally secondary in another situation. Moreover, the same persons and the same couple's attitudes may vary considerably over time while some of their basic qualities (like position in the life cycle, the stage of the relationship, relationship with the body, or expectations from the relationship) hardly change. More fundamentally, we can ask ourselves about the epistemological sense and practical pertinence of such an ambitious undertaking with regard to AIDS prevention. The hope of building a precise cause-and-effect model seems impossible in a field characterized by a great diversity of complex situations, where the stage is set with many variations in conduct and behaviour. For example, the slightest event (such as the impression of perceiving reluctance on the part of the partner) may destroy the strongest resolve (such as to use a condom) in a split second.

This conviction has been reinforced by research that has confirmed the central importance of the relationship in understanding attitudes toward the risk of HIV infection. We have seen, for example, that sexual partners' initial goals are never to protect themselves from AIDS. However, they are, at least generally, to share affection and pleasure. The way of protecting oneself from AIDS may constitute a resource for the development of the relationship. This changes the usual prevention perspective considerably. Taking the relationship to be a central reality implies, *de facto*, the recognition of the semi-arbitrary, even versatile nature of attitudes toward the risk. The complexity of and difficulty linked to the necessary consideration of the relationship challenge the very possibility of creating a theoretical model and explaining its epistemological nature with a view to practical applications.

The fact that we do not feel capable (or even see the sense) of connecting these factors in a stable way does not preclude these factors being relevant, and we feel that progress has been made by defining them, making them operational and understanding their influence. For example, it now seems certain that the stage of the relationship usually plays a crucial role, since sexual relationships change over time. Another example is the distinction between primary and secondary space and the tension that exists between them that enable us to shed light on some observations (for example, of relational norms) that would otherwise be extremely difficult to interpret. As work continues, the instruments of understanding behaviour may be refined and demonstrate their relevance without it being necessary to link them in a stable way. It would appear to be a matter of showing how the different factors selected may be composed in different ways according to the different situations and thus raise different questions about prevention. Building typologies is one of the methodologies that allow one to carry through and structure such work (Peto, *et al.*, 1992).

What is the practical relevance of this research? First, it may help leaders to design preventive measures in a knowledgeable way. The research as conceived here enables us to identify and understand problematic situations, to specify certain conditions for the possibility and success of preventive actions, to correct overly simplistic or preconceived ideas and to understand better people's points of view and the complex interaction between partners. If the research resulted in the recognition of complexity, that would be a considerable accomplishment. However, this research may also be used by the sexual partners themselves. It may help them understand better the situations in which they themselves are involved and the results of their own behaviour. This would be the purpose of developing a typology which presented situations, characteristics and conceptual sources for understanding them that would enable each person to situate him- or herself and recognize better by a proximity–distance game the singularity of his or her own situation The researcher's central, and fundamental, role is thus that of naming things and thereby enabling the recognition process to occur.

Note

1   The first assumption regarding the importance of the relationship was directly inspired by research recently done by the two teams who collaborated on this text, Peto, *et al.* (1992), in Belgium; and Bastard and Cardia-Vonèche (1992) in France and Switzerland. The second part of the assumption concerning the relationship with the body was studied by the French-Swiss team only.

References

BASTARD, B. and CARDIA-VONÈCHE, L. (with the participation of Mazoyer, M.) (1992) *Les choix et les comportements affectifs et sexuels face au sida. Une étude sociologique auprès de personnes séparées ou divorcées*, Paris: Centre de sociologie des organisations.

BOLTANSKI, L. (1968) *La découverte de la maladie*, Paris: Centre de sociologie de l'enseignement et de la culture, Maison des sciences de l'Homme.

BOURDIEU, P. (1972) 'Les stratégies matrimoniales dans le système de reproduction', *Annales*, **4–5**, juillet-octobre, pp. 1.105–1.126.

CARDIA-VONÈCHE, L., VON ALLMEN, M. and BASTARD, B. (1987) 'Fonctionnement familial et rapport à la santé: Essai d'analyse typologique', *Revue internationale d'action communautaire*, **18** (58), pp. 67–77.

DODIER, N. (1986) 'Corps fragiles. La construction sociale des événements corporels dans les activités quotidiennes du travail', *Revue française de sociologie*, **XXVII**, pp. 603–28.

GAGNON, J.H. and SIMON, W. (1986) 'Sexual scripts: Permanence and change', *Archives of Sexual Behaviour*, **15** (2), pp. 97–129.

GOFFMAN, E. (1974) *Les rites d'interaction*, Paris: Edition de Minuit.

HUSTON, T.L. and LEVINGER, G. (1978) 'Interpersonal attraction and relationship', *Annual Review of Psychology*, **29**, pp. 115–56.

KELLERHALS, J. and MONTANDON, C. (1991) *Les stratégies éducatives des familles, milieu social, dynamique familiale et éducation des pré-adolescents*, Paris: Delachaux et Nestlé.

LEVI-MAKARIUS, L. (1974) *Le sacré et la violation des interdits*, Paris: Payot.

OSIEK-PARISOD, F. (1990) *C'est bon pour ta santé! Représentations et pratiques familiales en matière d'éducation à la santé*, Genève: Cahier n° 31 du service de la recherche sociologique.

PADIOLEAU, J. (1986) *L'ordre social. Principes d'analyse sociologique*, Paris: L'Harmattan.

PETO, D., REMY, J., VAN CAMPENHOUDT, L. and HUBERT, M. (1992) *Sida: l'amour face à la peur*, Paris: L'Harmattan.

PIERRET, J. (1984) 'Les significations sociales de la santé: Paris, l'Essone, l'Hérault', in AUGÉ, M. and HERZLICH, C. *Le sens du mal, anthropologie, histoire, sociologie de la maladie*, Paris: Editions des archives contemporaines, pp. 217–56.

REISS, I.L. (1986a) 'A sociological journey into sexuality', *Journal of Marriage and the Family*, **48**, pp. 233–42.

REISS, I.L. (1986b) *Journey into Sexuality: An Exploratory Voyage*, New York: Prentice-Hall.

REMY, J. and VOYÉ, L. (1981) *Ville, ordre et violence*, Paris: PUF, Espace et Liberté.

TROUTOT, P.-Y. and MONTANDON, C. (1988) 'Systèmes d'action familiaux, attitudes éducatives et rapport à l'école: Une mise en perspective typologique', in PERRENOUD, P. and MONTANDON, C. (Eds) *Qui maîtrise l'école?*, Lausanne: Réalités Sociales, pp. 133–53.

VON ALLMEN, M., BASTARD, B. and CARDIA-VONÈCHE, L. (1987) 'Espaces sociaux, temps de l'échange et rapports familiaux: Une perspective typologique' in BAWIN-LEGROS, B. (Ed.) *Actes du colloque «La dynamique familiale et les constructions sociales du temps»*, Liège: Université de Liège, pp. 121–64.

VON ALLMEN, M., BASTARD, B., CARDIA-VONÈCHE, L. and LANGUIN, N. (1989) 'Les représentations de la santé dans la famille: Une analyse exploratoire', in D'HOUTAUD, A., FIELD, M. and GUEGUEN, R. (Eds) *Les représentations de la santé: bilan actuel, nouveaux développements*, colloque INSERM, Paris: Editions INSERM, pp. 297–312.

VON ALLMEN, M., BASTARD, B. and CARDIA-VONÈCHE, L. (1993) 'Les Femmes Divorcées et Le Sida: Celles qui Ferment Les Yeux et Celles qui Les Ouvrent', *Dialogue*, **121**, pp. 70–81.

Interaction and Risk-related Behaviour: Theoretical and Heuristic Landmarks

Luc Van Campenhoudt and Mitchell Cohen

Introduction

The preceding three chapters are united by the desire to take interactional processes, especially the relationship between partners, as the main focus of analysis. However, several different paths are taken from this common starting point as the authors answer questions such as: What is the exact nature of the interactions that we want to study? What are the links between the dyadic relationships between partners and the relationship's social environment? How can we distinguish between the relationship itself and the partners' involvement in the relationship? How can the interactional process best be conceptualized with regard to AIDS prevention?

This chapter consists of two parts. Part one analyses and discusses solutions proposed by the four theoretical approaches presented in the preceding chapters, i.e., 1) social systems; 2) social network; 3) cognitive and social psychology; 4) sociology of social relationships. This analysis will discuss the following elements for each theoretical perspective: basic assumptions and key research questions; their use of causal models and the types of explanation from which they are derived; their scopes and how they are implemented (their operationalization). The second part examines how the various approaches allow for the main dimensions of the relationships to be taken into account. These dimensions include situational, temporal, meaning, power, emotional, and risk status factors. Throughout the chapter we identify various problems and failings and search for ways to overcome them.

Theoretical Constructions of Interactional Processes

Systems Theory

Drawing upon Luhmann's theories, Ahlemeyer perceives the relationships between two partners to be a dyadic system of intimate communication. One of the basic assumptions of the social systems theory is the autonomy and internal self-organization of the system. The system's basic building blocks are communications between partners. They are highly temporal events, for new situations are created from moment to moment. Still, to limit their own indetermination these systems develop specific structures, thereby separating themselves from other systems.

The distinctive unity of intimate systems lies in their focus on sexual interactions. Ahlemeyer classifies sexual interactions into four categories – romantic, hedonistic, matrimonial and prostitutive – each of which is governed by its own logic and internal dynamics. Each system has its own rules for communication and reciprocal expectations that structure the partners' interactions. In this approach, the actors' behaviours are elements of the system. To use these systems in designing prevention strategies, each researcher must answer the following key questions: What type of system is involved? How does it reproduce itself and develop its autonomy? How does protected sex occur in such a system?

The systems theory is built on a consistent logical foundation that adds insights into some key questions about sexual behaviour and HIV/AIDS prevention. For example, the systems analysis focuses not so much on how the system is influenced by its social environment but, on the contrary, how the intimate system develops and achieves a specific identity apart from its environment. Systems theory establishes the hypothesis that each system defines the conditions under which it accepts to be influenced by its environment according to its own logic and norms of operation.

With regard to intimate systems, we can deduce from Ahlemeyer's chapter that, first, all intimate systems are defined in contrast to daily life. For example, nudity and intimate physical contact are not usually part of one's daily work schedule or visits with friends and acquaintances. Second, each intimate system develops its own logics with different implications for prevention. For example, the romantic system involves the creation by the partners of a sentimental universe whereby the couple close the system on itself with a disregard for the future. The relationship is based on codes of communication that must manifest reciprocal trust and admiration. Under these conditions, risk-taking may be prized as a way of showing one's bond, and a set of communication codes gradually turns into rituals in which condom use may become very difficult and unlikely. In contrast to the disregard for the future, the matrimonial system is built upon long-term plans of raising a family. Using a condom in a matrimonial system with a high value of fidelity and trust means that the spouse who has extramarital affairs may find him or herself in a very awkward situation, where condom use is interpreted as infidelity rather than birth control. The hedonistic system focuses on satisfying one's sexual desires. Pleasure, whimsy, creativity, and immediacy predominate over other concerns, although birth control and protection against HIV infection are often practices which preserve the ability to continue hedonistic behaviours. The prostitutive system focuses on the nature of the buyer–seller relationship and explicit negotiation over sexual activity, including HIV/AIDS prevention.

The systems theory as developed by Luhmann and applied to sexual relationships by Ahlemeyer is a functional as well as systemic explanation. Systemic explanation is usually considered to have the following characteristics (see Berthelot, 1990; Franck, 1994):

- Reciprocal causality between the interacting components. The components behave differently than in other relationships, otherwise their behaviour would be independent from the relationship being considered.
- The parts being arranged in a special configuration.
- Self-organization, which leads to its conservation and relatively closed boundaries.
- The constant transformation of relationships amongst the components according to internal laws where the system's conservation is ensured by the constant transformation of its internal relations.
- A hierarchy of levels, from the most complex to the simplest.

Luhmann's theory combines systemic and functional explanations to the extent that instances of communication between the partners are explained by their functions in the system's scheme of self-reproduction. For the functional explanation, the needs of the whole system are what oblige its components to carry out a given function. As a result, the system's dynamics may be depicted as a spiral. All of the communications that constitute the system generate the system's laws of self-(re)production – the rules of the game. In return, these rules determine the network of possible communications.

This is an example of formal causality, in which the theory strives to reveal the dynamic laws that the phenomena under study are supposed to obey. The laws of the system must be considered to be a structure that determines a field of belonging and all the processes that occur in this field. For example, in a prostitutive system the prostitute and client bargain over a price and what they will do together, but the rules that govern the communication do not say what will actually happen between them. For this, one must specify the conditions and actual circumstances in which the system is called into play. These conditions cannot be accounted for through a dynamic law (Ladrière, 1994). In the above situation, for example, these are the specific expectations of each client, the price he is willing to pay, the amount of time available to him, how attracted he may be to a particular prostitute, the fact that this is their first encounter or, on the contrary, he is a steady client, and a string of haphazard events that are part of their relationship's context. In short, a systems perspective is never entirely determinant and does not allow prediction of a specific behaviour. Instead, it determines a field of probabilities, for instance, if there is penetration, the partners will probably use a condom. As we have seen, the main task of the researcher who wants to develop such dynamic laws thus becomes to delineate their scopes as accurately as possible. Ahlemeyer, for example, tries to attach specific logics to his four types of intimate systems.

This gives rise to a number of points concerning this theory's relevance for understanding HIV/AIDS risk-related behaviour. The first point concerns the advantages of examining the entire set of sexual relations from a systemic point of view. In the area of sex, the first difficulty is that the situations under study are highly variable and volatile. Some of them, such as what happens in a brothel or on the wedding night in a traditional society, may be highly structured in that they follow a relatively predetermined pattern that is governed by easily identifiable, binding rules. Others, such as chance encounters between relative strangers, take place in a framework in which norms are less structured and blurrier. In this case, the formal model may not explain behaviour very well. Sociologists who study systems may say that even informal relationships are governed by specific types of logic (social codes governing encounters, seduction–courtship rituals, etc.), and that the strength of an analysis is precisely to go beyond the illusion of spontaneity in sexual and love relationships to reveal the underlying communication structures. A second difficulty is that when it comes to sex, many encounters have unclear borders. This makes the decision about the type of system to which they belong difficult. The partners' respective expectations may be, to a large extent, undetermined, different, even opposed to each other. For example, one partner's expectations may centre on elements of the matrimonial system whereas the other partner's expectations revolve around elements of the hedonistic system.

The preceding theoretical clarification gives us some clues as to how to implement the systems theory in actual research. Once the field or fields of application of the phenomena being studied and consequently the type or types of systems involved have been determined, the aim is to understand *why* the behaviour or phenomena, for example, taking a risk or using a condom, occurred. This is done using structures that characterize each system. Since these structures define the rules in the field being considered, the goal of the empirical work is, according to Franck (1994), to check whether the phenomena that are observed in a given field can all be deduced from the hypothetical structures that define and circumscribe these phenomena's field of belonging. To achieve this goal, it is no longer a matter of increasing the number of observations to check frequencies or patterns, but to diversify them in order to induce the common structure that shapes all these observations.

In discovering more and more accurately the structure in question, one concomitantly improves understanding of the observed phenomena.

The systems theory is widely accepted as being remarkably consistent and, as shown in the second part of this chapter, it allows for the widest range of phenomena. A criticism of systemic and functionalist theories concerns the actors' status and the meaning they give to their experiences, and some will feel that there are better approaches for understanding sexual behaviour. Regardless of one's belief in this perspective, it brings many heuristic resources from which pertinent research questions may be asked.

Social Network Theory

Ferrand and Snijders, for their part, consider the relationship between partners to be part of a social network. Each partner effectively has a set of interpersonal relations, some of which are sexual or potentially sexual. According to the normative network perspective, the part of the network that is composed of relations with significant others is most important for understanding AIDS risk-related behaviour. Each individual tends to seek the approval and fear the disapproval of those whose opinions are valued. In fact, according to normative network theory, there are no norms without effective social control through the social environment. Thus, it is not enough that such norms be proclaimed officially by the significant others; the norms must actually correspond to reality. So, for example, in some professional circles marital fidelity is the stated norm, but everyone knows that many colleagues have at least one extramarital partner. In that instance, provided that the affair is kept discreet, the norm is not actually fidelity but the right to have other partners. Such are some of the basic assumptions of the normative network theory applied to sexual behaviour.

To understand the sexual partners' behaviour, one must then answer the following key questions: Who are the significant others who count with regard to the behaviour being studied (in this case, who count in the various types of behaviour that make up a sexual relationship)? What are these significant others' effective norms? What behaviours will be approved or disapproved of by the significant others?

Ferrand and Snijders note the other functions of the social network when thinking in terms of designing prevention campaigns: 1) it is the relay for and way of personalizing public campaign messages; 2) it constitutes the market of potential sexual partners; and 3) it is the channel of information about personal life. Moreover, the social network theory is an analytical framework that allows several aspects of the relationship to be better understood. Thus, for example, an investigator who uses the resources of social network theory will posit that the balance of power between partners depends primarily on the possibility of alternative partners, that is, the respective networks' compositions.

The social network-based approach to AIDS risk-related sexual behaviour has very different basic assumptions, key questions and key concepts from the systems approach. However, the two approaches rely basically on formal causality. For social network theory, this enables one to reconstitute the configurations of the networks in which the relationship being studied takes place and determine the logics from which possible, even probable (if one is optimistic) behaviour may be deduced. For example, Ferrand and Snijders hypothesize that the more homogeneous a network is, the more powerful its influences on the norms governing the relationship are. Here we find the main features of systemic causality, i.e., reciprocal causality between interacting elements that make up a particular configuration, self-organization, and ranked levels (networks and sub-networks, etc.) that likewise interact with each other.

Still, according to Ferrand and Snijders, whereas social network theory can shed considerable light on how a sexual relationship unfolds, it cannot account for the relationship's own dynamics. Each relationship is a singular reality in itself, a specific temporal process composed of bargaining and agreements that often change over time. That is why our authors also support the relational theory paradigm, which they contrast with the *focal actor* theory.

Nevertheless, through their insistence on taking the configuration of social networks and the specific nature and dynamics of each relationship into account jointly, these authors stress the need for a connection between formal and material causality. In particular, the informal way in which material causality accounts for the internal dynamics of sexual relationships complements the formal, structural, social networks approach and helps us understand why only some of the wide range of behaviours that the configuration of the partners' networks authorizations occur. In so doing, these authors imply that the systemic explanation must be supplemented by an actancial explanation. In the latter type of explanation, a phenomenon such as behaviour towards the risk of HIV/AIDS does not result from systems or structures that exist independently from the partners, even though the latter help renew them, but from the partners' own decisions, actions and interactions. Actions taken by social actors who are involved with others in social relationships constantly define and redefine the broader social context. From this point of view, systems and contexts are nothing more than the state of social relationships, at a given time, which exist alone and thus must be the foci of analysis. This is further discussed in the introduction to Section III.

Cognitive and Social Psychology

Ludwig's approach differs from the previous two approaches in several respects. Most importantly, unlike systems and social network theories, material causality plays the major role in Ludwig's approach.

According to Ludwig, the concepts of social psychology have evolved over the past few years and give added insights into sexual behaviour between partners. In Ludwig's point of view it is the individuals' involvement in their relationships in specific contexts and situations that is the focus of the analysis rather than the relationships themselves. She thus discusses four dimensions of the individuals' involvement in the relationship. The first one is the way individuals build their perceptions, especially of risks and the relationship in which they are, or plan to be, involved. This is a traditional concern of social psychology and is found in individual-based models such as the Health Belief Model – although Ludwig believes that such models would benefit from added attention to the individual's likes and dislikes. The second dimension is the social nature of individuals, where they are socialized and interact with others. Placing individuals in a social perspective is accompanied by a shift in the way individual perceptions are conceptualized. Social psychologists speak less of *thinking* and *understanding* and more about *meanings* and *significance*; for example, what does it mean to tell the other person: 'I am thinking about the disease' or 'I want to have safer sex'? The question of meaning goes beyond the consideration of isolated individuals; the cultural, historical and anthropological dimensions take on added significance. The third dimension is taking actual contexts and situations into account so that the Who? questions of traditional social psychology are replaced by When? questions, e.g., When do people perceive risks or try to forget their existence? When do people take risks readily or try to protect themselves? When are people's attempts successful? The fourth dimension concerns the phases of the relationship, for the partners' involvement in the relationship and the norms governing their relationship change with the phases.

The basic assumption of Ludwig's approach is that the course of a sexual relationship and AIDS risk-related reactions within this relationship depend on how the partners are involved in the relationship. Although the interacting individuals are determined by culture and are defined as social individuals, Ludwig's approach relies mainly on actancial and hermeneutic explanations. The hermeneutic approach is characterized by the search for the significance of human behaviours and reveals the *signified* from a set of *signifiers* by means of which they can be understood. For the cognitive social psychologist, key questions are: What are the partners' perceptions of their relationship and what meaning does it have for them? How are these perceptions and meaning influenced by the partners' social and cultural conditions? What are the links between these perceptions and meaning and the actual context of their relationship, the situation in which they are involved and the phase of their relationship?

It appears that two axes for operationalization may be deducted from Ludwig's communication. Firstly the hermeneutic approach entails the use of intensive, fairly unguided methods. The idea is to allow the people whose behaviour is being studied to express themselves rather freely and to establish connections between the signifier, as the material expression of meaning, and the signified, as the contents of meanings. Second, the material causality point of view means, as Ludwig states very clearly, that a careful, detailed description of the situation and what occurs between partners is required. Such a material model will be pertinent if, with the help of empirical data, it fits the process of what is actually happening (Franck, 1994). Such an approach has an extremely broad scope, since the proposed categories may apply to all individuals and all types of sexual relationships and do not presuppose laws of formal theoretical structures, which are neither universal nor timeless.

Relational Sociology

Bastard and his team from France and Switzerland and Peto and her team from Brussels try to find a common denominator that enables them to connect their qualitative data that was collected using diverging epistemological and theoretical presuppositions. Bastard, *et al.*, study the influences of various sociological factors that are important for understanding behaviour in response to the risk of sexual transmission of HIV/AIDS. The relationship is the main focus of their analysis. That is why their approach has been dubbed *relational sociology*. The factors are the type of involvement in the relationship (fusion or association), the stage of the relationship (courtship–seduction, familiarity, or unravelling), the relationship's social area (primary or secondary), the balance of power between the partners (determined by their economic, social, cultural and symbolic resources), and the relationship with the body and health management (instrumental or reflexive).

These factors are not linked to each other in a consistent theory; they are simply juxtaposed. The authors' intention is not to develop a scheme of formal causality like those of the systems and social network theories. Such an attempt was invalidated when they tried to test hypotheses built on a linear, binary, cause-and-effect relationship, such as the hypotheses that condoms would be used more frequently in fusion relationships and when partners have reflexive relationships with the body than when they have an instrumental relationship with the body. The result of their work is to provide conceptual resources from which it becomes possible to define, in an orderly and relevant manner, the actual situations and problems that arise in each situation with regard to AIDS. In so doing, they are closer to Ludwig's objectives. For example, a given situation may be defined by two inexperienced partners of the same social status, one involved fusionally and the other instrumentally in the unravelling phase of a primary relationship. The subject of inquiry becomes the impact of these situational factors on their sexual behaviour.

This approach uses material explanations. The conceptual categories used to describe actual situations are drawn from their qualitative research and the work of others, such as Gagnon and Simon's (1986). From these, we know it is important to take into account one or the other aspect of the problem (such as the phase of the relationship and the partners' positions in their life cycles) because they render the situation intelligible with regard to the stated problem. Elements of formal theories are used to grasp as correctly as possible the factual conditions of the relationship. The diversity of theories means that several causal explanations could be used, such as structural, hermeneutic, and actancial. There is no general rule for material causality-oriented approaches. Instead there is a need for flexibility where different components are assigned degrees of importance depending on the situation. A factor that is highly relevant in one case may be unimportant in other cases and vice versa. So, for example, gender-based power may carry great weight in some societies and social networks but much less weight in others.

What we said about operationalizing the previous approach also applies to this one. Let us simply add that this type of approach can lead to the development of typologies. One key concern is that the selection and arrangement of its criteria must not be so numerous as to reduce the advantages of categorization.

The Main Dimensions of the Relationship between Sexual Partners

In the first part of this chapter we compared the different interaction-oriented perspectives on their epistemological and theoretical foundations. In this part of the chapter we tackle the problem of theorizing the sexual interaction through its main dimensions. For each dimension, we shall elucidate the resources (research questions, hypotheses, etc.) proposed by each theoretical perspective and discuss them with a critical spirit. We shall also identify the problems for which these approaches do not offer adequate solutions. This discussion provides an heuristic device for further research.

The Situational Dimension of the Sexual Relationship

The context in which a sexual relationship takes places exerts a decisive influence over the relationship's course and the partners' behaviour. In the preceding chapters some authors see a network in a physical and temporal substratum whereas others will see a system. Ludwig contends that the context's influence can be circumscribed by *when* questions, for example: When do people perceive or try to forget risks? According to Ludwig, the material conditions of the places or times are used to describe the context (e.g., the bedroom Sunday morning, a beach on a summer's day, a romantic restaurant in the evening, a sauna, etc.) and are of interest because they constitute the physical substratum of the partners' involvement. Bastard, *et al.*, take context into account. The concept of primary and secondary space imply some interaction between space–time (downtown, in the evening) and the nature of the partners' involvement (an anonymous one-night stand), in which the material component plays an active part by inducing behaviour and communication codes with which the partners tend to attribute natural behaviours. In Ahlemeyer's writings, the material conditions of space and time are linked to the structure of the communications that make up intimate systems. As we have seen, systems analysis requires that the various systems and their scopes be differentiated from the start, prior to empirical analysis. In Ferrand and Snijders' logic of network analysis, each context is a particular arrangement of the partners' social networks. So, for example, sauna encounters may be considered to form a narrow, closed, monofunctional network with its own norms that is protected from negative sanctions by significant others who are in other, non-overlapping networks.

In general, we believe it is worthwhile to raise the status of material conditions. The sociological notion of the *milieu* that has been developed by Durkheim and others might be extremely useful, especially from the systems analysis point of view.

The Temporal Dimension of the Sexual Relationship

Social scientists have traditionally studied social phenomena more in terms of their structures than in terms of their temporal dimensions. As Ferrand and Snijders stress, devising a theory to connect these two dimensions is a difficult problem. That is why they chose to limit themselves to developing a middle-range theory that covers well-circumscribed research questions.

For Ahlemeyer, on the contrary, it seems that the systems theory claims to integrate the temporal or dynamic dimension into the structural dimension. Indeed, the system is composed of communications that consist of highly temporalized events that constantly modify the system's very structure. On the other hand, the system's structure determines subsequent communication, so that the system replicates itself due to the fact that its components are constantly changing. However, each type of intimate system follows its own logic, and researchers can anticipate certain behaviours. In his text Ahlemeyer does not provide details about his operationalization. Does the formal theory of systems itself contain the means to proceed farther along this path, and just how far? Mustn't it be combined with other types of explanation, say, actancial or hermeneutic (since it is hard to see how the meaning the actors give to their experiences would not be taken into account here)?

Bastard, *et al.*, operationalize the temporal dimension of the relationship by incorporating temporal phases (courtship–seduction, familiarity, and unravelling phases). According to several authors (Peto, 1992; Gagnon and Simon, 1986; Van Campenhoudt *et al.*, 1994) these phases may be the most decisive in determining risk behaviour. For example, some partners no longer use a condom after only three or four encounters because the partners quickly feel they know and trust each other. Ludwig also mentions this point. She suggests using the *scheme* and *script* concepts, which are defined as *cognitive expectations*. In a more relational or interactional perspective it might be possible to identify *interactional schemes* or *interactional scripts* in which different sequences could be partially stabilized by norms produced by the interaction, rituals or socially established habits. However, such schemes could also include key moments when multiple scenarios must be considered by the actors. The Social Exchange Theory developed by Emerson (1976), and Huston and Levinger (1978), and others, has already tried to identify comparable scripts. According to Deven and Meredith (Chapter 8), Gagnon's sexual script theory is a way to formalize and operationalize this kind of temporal influence.

In the interactional perspective advocated throughout the book, the relationship's dynamics and outcome are basically the results of a bargaining process between the partners over time. The relationship's temporality combines with yet other temporalities, such as generation effects, changes in the institutional framework (preventive measures, etc.), the course of the epidemic, the partner's position in their respective life course, etc. This further complicates the question of the relationship's dynamics. As Cohen and Hubert's text will show, factors related to risk-related behaviour vary within different temporal contexts. In Chapter 9, Guizzardi, Stella and Remy evoke a dialectic dimension of social phenomena. Thus, contradictions between two or more elements of social reality (such as between messages in the media) are unavoidable and create a dynamic process of tension, resolution of tension, new tension, and so forth. Sexual relations and risk-related behaviour offer a particularly fertile ground for dialectic explanations, which consider a phenomenon to be 'a moment in a process of becoming' (Berthelot, 1990). In such an approach the behaviour under study is not considered the culmination of a process but a stage in the partners' relationship. Determining the temporal aspects is an important dimension of understanding behaviour.

Meaning of the Relationship

As Ludwig has shown, an interaction-based approach calls for switching from thinking to meaning. To understand behaviour the crucial information is no longer the partners' knowledge about AIDS and how they describe themselves but determining the meaning of different communications and behaviours in the relationship. Ludwig will wonder, for example, what it means to say to the other person, 'I am thinking about the disease' or 'I want to have safer sex'. This point of view is firmly supported by Bastard *et al.*, whose research shows that ways of adapting to risk can be considered expressions of relational significance. Proposing or not proposing a condom can be interpreted as a message of intention, and the use (or non-use) of the condom is translated by the partners to communicate something else, such as how much the other partner is valued. For prevention purposes this means that an effort should be made to give condoms a positive meaning, for example, to get their use to be interpreted as having respect for one's partner.

Ferrand and Snijder's consideration of meanings is limited to references to the media's influence. They emphasize how the media's messages are interpreted by opinion leaders within the social network. Perception of risk is a consequence of the interplay of the interpretations of messages by the actors in the network: the media, opinion leaders, friends, partners and the individual.

In Ahlemeyer's approach, it is not the meanings themselves that are taken into account, but rather the fact that some things are said between partners and other things are not. The idea in itself is interesting, for a social system rests upon a consensus about which messages of communication are acceptable and which are not. For example, a romantic intimate system based on blind trust may ban speaking about condoms, because, by definition, they represent a practical concern outside the system's boundary. Deven and Meredith (Chapter 8) and Guizzardi, Stella and Remy (Chapter 9) will point out the ideological and social nature of perceptions of sexual experiences. Their meanings are the social product of transactions between actors, regardless of the level involved (macrosocial, microsocial or relational). Meanings conferred on a relationship are not produced by a process external to the relationship; they are produced by the relationship and its interactions.

Power in the Sexual Relationship

An interactional approach that did not take the partner's balance of power into account would be built on the erroneous illusion of an equal relationship, like a game of chance in which the participants all start off with exactly the same odds. There are a number of reasons to consider balances of power when trying to understand sexual behaviour. First of all, they are inherent in sexual relationships, which bring together partners who pursue different objectives with unequal resources. Next, the influence of the partners' respective social positions on the course of the relationship occurs mainly at this level. Finally, this is the dimension that is the most deeply influenced by institutional and macrosocial factors such as gender roles and gender-based power relationships, kinship systems, and the sexual ideologies that are established for an entire society or a social class. A theoretical perspective that focuses on the dyadic relationship requires an understanding of how partners use resources in their relationships.

Using Pierre Bourdieu's theory about capital, Bastard, *et al.*, divide the resources available to partners into four types, each affecting the balance of power (Peto, *et al.*, 1992). The first category, social resources, consists of social networks that the partners can mobilize to achieve their ends. As Ferrand and Meredith argue, from the network analysis standpoint the balance of power between partners depends on the availability of alternative sexual partners or network. The second category, economic resources, suggests that those with economic resources have various advantages, such as the dependence of the partner without economic resources and increased opportunities for meeting people through travel and increased mobility. The third category consists of cultural resources, which are acquired through education and experience. Culture dictates the values assigned to family, fertility, beauty, youthfulness, and sex appeal. Cohen and Hubert suggest in Chapter 11 that partners are in a much stronger position when they bring strongly held cultural values to a relationship. When one partner brings strong cultural values to a relationship, he or she is in a more powerful position to dictate sexual behaviour. Finally, the fourth category consists of symbolic resources. These refer to the ability to acquire a certain status or attractiveness in the eyes of potential or actual partners. They are usually derived from the ability to exploit the preceding three types of resources, such as the prestige or sex appeal associated with wealth, social status, beauty or fertility.

Explaining the balance of power between partners can be facilitated by comparing the social, economic, cultural and symbolic resources in a relationship. For example, men often have greater economic and physical resources than women, although the degrees and forms will vary from one society to the next. To conceptualize the influence of gender-based power on HIV/AIDS risk-related behaviour we must delve deeper into gender studies and investigate the relationships between factors related to gender-based power, such as physical violence, economic need, discrimination, and reproduction.

It is not surprising that Ahlemeyer sees the problem of gender-based power as differing from one system to the other and Ferrand and Snijders speak about bargaining. Transaction and negotiation take place with variable intensities in each specific situation. For example, to use the language of social systems theory, we could say that negotiation is part of a prostitutive system and safer sex is likely to be discussed, since it is important to the self-preservation of the system. In a romantic system the partner voicing the values of trust and intimacy, which are frequently related negatively to condom use, is much more likely to be dominant. In both cases the partners are involved in a process of variable length during which they try to achieve their ends, to adjust to each other and to find *modi vivendi* that depend basically on the balance of power that develops between them. This means that one must look at each specific instance of how macrosocially-determined imbalances in resources and power are used in microsocial processes. Even if a balance of power is unequal, the dominated partner is seldom completely defenceless and may even be dominant with regard to certain aspects of the relationship. There is much work to be done in providing an analytical framework that allows an understanding of the role power plays in the partners' interactions. Deven and Meredith in Chapter 8 discuss the effect of macrosocial elements on the power relationship.

The Emotional Dimensions of the Sexual Relationship

Emotions are part of a sexual relationship and, as Ludwig notes, are strongly related to AIDS risk-related behaviour. Some of the following chapters discuss the emotional elements more than the previous three. At this point, we note that emotions can have a key or peripheral position in the relationship, be its main objective, or serve another end. We must guard against unequivocal, simplistic points of view that create a false conflict between emotion and rationality.

The Status of Risk in Sexual Relationships

There is a simplistic, wrong impression that an individual is constantly battling the temptations of passion and desire on one hand and reasonableness of protecting him or herself from the risk of HIV contamination on the other. Our authors counter this image with another one, namely, that risk-taking is not irrational but helps constitute the meaning and function of the relationship. It has been shown, for example, that the deliberate refusal to use a condom may be a way to consolidate a relationship or that the attraction of a secondary relationship that escapes the usual forms of social control may be all the more necessary if the primary relationship is highly structured and does not satisfy a particular sexual need.

These examples depart from a romantic view of risk, whereby some individuals, even most individuals, are basically irrational all or part of the time, as if they were possessed by overwhelming forces. The contributors to this book say little about death wishes or fascination with death, as a psychoanalyst might. Without denying the benefit of psychoanalysis to explain deviant behaviour, we find that behaviour associated with the risk of being infected with HIV is part of a normal experience from the standpoint of both statistics and norms. It is part of trying to bind a partner to oneself, looking for sexual satisfaction, putting up a good show, making some secondary space for one-self outside the usual areas of social control, finding the right answers to un-foreseen developments, and feeling at ease with one's close friends or relatives. In the great majority of cases, the demands of a fulfilling personal and social life are what lead people to engage in risky behaviour that is qualified as irrational only by those who are blinded by technocratic logic (as discussed in some detail by Guizzardi in Chapter 12).

The acceptance of risk obviously complicates matters for prevention. Prevention strategies should focus on the interactional process, and under-standing the risk-taking dimension of sexual relationships can make it pos-sible to gauge the probability of success of preventive efforts. Ferrand and Snijder's suggestion to promote talking about sex seems simple but, as one qualitative investigation conducted in Belgium revealed, some respondents would not dare suggest using condoms to their partners but would, neverthe-less, like their partners to suggest using condoms and, if their partners did so, would then see them as decent people who do not shirk their respon-sibilities. With regard to the issue of risk-taking in secondary spaces, initiatives such as campaigns to promote the use of condoms in brothels have signifi-cant and rapid results, whereas working on partners' emotional structures will mean a long-term and expensive counselling effort. Finally, taking the risk of the relationship into account leads one to believe that widespread *zero risk* or *safe sex* is not a reasonable goal. Sights should doubtless be set on a viable balance founded on a combination of community measures and the exercise of individual responsibility to strive for safer sex. Generally speaking, today's theoretical approaches are directed more toward explaining unsafe behaviour, which is not the same as developing protocols for behaviour change or main-taining safer sex.

The next section of this book discusses why we have moved from the individual-oriented perspectives to interaction-oriented perspectives. Our efforts to organize the various theoretical approaches through comparison of their epistemological and theoretical foundations and to examine different ways to operationalize the main dimensions of the sexual relationship will continue in Chapter 7 by Bastard, *et al.*

References

BERTHELOT, J.-M. (1990) *L'intelligence du social*, Paris: PUF.
EMERSON, M. (1976) 'Social exchange theory', *Annual Review of Sociology*, **2**, pp. 335–63.
FRANCK, R. (Ed.) (1994) *Faut-il chercher aux causes une raison? L'explication causale dans les sciences humaines*, Paris: Institut interdisciplinaire d'études épistémologiques.

GAGNON, J.H. and SIMON W. (1986) 'Sexual scripts: Permanence and change', in *Archives of Sexual Behaviour*, **15** (2) pp. 97–129.

HUSTON, T.L. and LEVINGER, G. (1978) 'Interpersonal attraction and relationship', *Annual Review of Psychology*, **29**, pp. 115–56.

LADRIÈRE, J. (1994) 'La causalité dans les sciences de la nature et dans les sciences humaines', in FRANCK, R. *Faut-il chercher aux causes une raison? L'explication causale dans les sciences humaines*, Paris: Institut interdisciplinaire d'études épistémologiques, pp. 248–74.

PETO, D., REMY, J., VAN CAMPENHOUDT, L. and HUBERT, M. (1992) *Sida, l'amour face à la peur*, Paris: L'Harmattan.

VAN CAMPENHOUDT, L., REMY, J., PETO, D. and HUBERT, M. (1994) 'La relation sexuelle comme transaction sociale: À partir des réactions au risque du sida', in *Vie quotidienne et démocratie. Pour une sociologie de la transaction sociale (suite)*, Paris: L'Harmattan, pp. 93–112.

Section II

From Individual to Interaction

Introduction

The interaction-based perspectives presented in the first part of this book are in contrast to approaches that use an individual's attitudes, beliefs, knowledge, and social characteristics as predictors of sexual behaviour. This second part of the book is devoted to a critical discussion of these individual-oriented perspectives. Far from systematically exploring all the variations and aspects of individual-oriented models, the critiques presented by the following authors facilitate understanding sexual behaviour based on partner and peer interactions.

It is with this mindset that we suggest reading the next three chapters. In the first two chapters Ingham and van Zessen and Moatti, Hausser and Agrafiotis base their criticism on logical arguments and use their own research findings to establish a few reference points for interaction-oriented approaches. In the third chapter Bastard and Cardia-Vonèche summarize the debate on the individual's rationality and suggest thinking in terms of the 'rationality of the relationship'. In this review they refer to the two preceding chapters, but also to other texts in the first part of this book, especially those of Ahlemeyer and Ludwig and Bastard *et al.*

In the following chapters, there are two fundamental criticisms of individual-based approaches. The first is epistemological and concerns the type of explanation on which these approaches rely. The second questions the theoretical base of the individual-oriented perspectives.

Correlation and Explanation

One of the most serious criticisms of individual-oriented models made by the authors is that, in testing such models, researchers often turn sets of correlations into explanations. This criticism is found in other works (Wunsch, 1994; Boudon and Bourricaud, 1982). Boudon and Bourricaud (1982) write that a correlation cannot pass for an explanation, regardless of the intensity of the correlation, for the logic of the individual actions that underlies the correlation has to be revealed. Ingham and van Zessen expand on this criticism. They refute an explanation for behaviour that is based on a series of cause-and-effect relationships. To explain human and social behaviour they say that one must grasp the *reasons* that people do what they do and take the processes of partner-to-partner interaction into account. Moatti, *et al.* acknowledge that the individual-oriented models have shown the importance of some contextual elements in determining behaviour, but they criticize these models for having turned these elements into explanations for why people take risks.

According to these authors, this explanatory shortfall stems from two reasons. First, they do not include the significance that the relationship has for each partners and the reality of the relationship itself. Second, the explanations are too mechanical and linear to explain human and social phenomena. This does not mean that the establishment of bivariate and/or multivariate correlations is of no use for these more complex models. On the contrary, such correlations can help build more comprehensive models. Specifically, they can help guide the search for the best forms of the processes being studied under a systemic or actancial approach. In exploring new avenues opened up by the expected usefulness theory, Moatti, Hausser and Agrafiotis, like other authors (Devillé, 1994), show that economics has already embarked on this path. They acknowledge the contributions made by various investigations, particularly some in North America, that have identified various variables that are systematically associated with a high probability of risk-taking. However, they criticize the fact that explanations are deduced strictly from the related factors. The need for explanations to go beyond the correlated variables is seen in the demographic work of Loriaux (1994). He notes, 'it is impossible to understand changes in a set of demographic phenomena and interpret their statistical interdependence correctly without repositioning them in the both overall and historical context of the system or systems to which they belong.' Similarly, in a systemic model a cause-and-effect relationship is interpreted as being a covariation between two elements of the system that are involved in a constant process of rebalancing due to contextual and environmental factors.

Franck (1994) suggests we should continue to search for empirical patterns, such as correlations, and use them to complement systemic, actancial or other types of explanations. Ingham and van Zessen, for example, find the reasons for sexual behaviour in the interaction of partners. Thus, if we systematically see greater exposure to risk after the break-up of a meaningful relationship, the statistical relationship between these two phenomena does not explain the exposure to risk. It is merely the starting point to help the investigator grasp what is going on in the individuals' lives and relationships that leads them to take greater risks. What is clear is that research into risk-related behaviour in sexual relationships can ill afford to rely on linear causality models, regardless of their degree of sophistication.

Ingham and van Zessen emphasize the futility of adding boxes to models in hopes of explaining more variance between variables when the model itself

is based on unsatisfactory presuppositions. They insist less on the need to predict sexual behaviour than on the usefulness of discovering the processes that
lead to different types of risk behaviour for HIV infection. This ties in with
some of the aspects developed in the first part of this book. For example, in
Chapter 4 Van Campenhoudt and Cohen showed that the relevance of a
theory is not measured by its predictive ability but rather, in the case of formal
theories, by its ability to reveal the logics behind phenomena and, in the case
of material theories, by how closely it fits reality.

From *Homo Oeconomicus* to *Homo Socialis*

The authors of all three chapters in this section conclude unanimously that
the rational individual paradigm is not suitable here. If we take the paradigm
to extremes, the rational individual or *Homo oeconomicus* compares all of the
risks and rewards that are possible in a given situation and take into account
all of what they consider to be the other actors' probable reactions for the
purpose of achieving the optimal effect for themselves. Thus, it is rational to
use a condom as protection from AIDS in potentially risky sex if individuals
are convinced of their own vulnerability. To alter risky behaviours individuals
must be provided with additional information about HIV's transmission routes,
means of protection, etc., and it is necessary to show them that their interest
lie in safer sex. Bastard and Cardia-Vonèche show in their review of the texts
that the conception of individual rationality can, of course, be enlarged to
consider the individual a complex being who changes according to circumstances, but even then they think that we would remain relatively helpless to
understand AIDS risk-related behaviour, for the actor would continue to be
considered an individual, in isolation from the actual interactions.

This image of the *rational individual* is not specific to individual-oriented
models. It is also found in models that focus directly on interaction processes. We saw the rational man in the first part of this book, in Ferrand and
Snijders' reference to Coleman's normative theory. According to this theory,
it is rational to comply with the effective norms of the group to which one
belongs, for that enables the individual to avoid sanctions. As the various
approaches rely on different presuppositions, this attempt runs into difficulties that Ferrand and Snijders identify and that are inherent in all new
attempts at conceptualization. Looking at the problem from a different angle,
we feel that the challenge is not so much the rationality of choice as that
individual-oriented models promote the idea that rational sexual decisions
are made alone. Instead, it is the contention of this section that there are
some cost/benefit calculations and an optimization of decision-making in
people's behaviour, but that is far from the only concern when it comes to
sex, especially if the activity carries a strong emotional charge.

The second main criticism of the individual-oriented theories is that they consider individuals *per se*, with their own (personal or social) characteristics, separate from the interactions in which they are involved. In this section the reader will note that most of the models that claim to be interaction-oriented do take the individual into account, but as a being who is incorporated in interpersonal interactions and whose interactive sexual behaviours constitute the relationship. This was explicit in Ludwig's remarks about the way partners commit themselves to a relationship; hence the importance that Ludwig attaches to the meanings that the partners give to their relationship and their experiences within the relationship. When Bastard and Cardia-Vonèche study the influences of the types of fusion or associative involvement in a relationship they take the same point of view. From this perspective the interaction is nothing more than all of the partners' interactive behaviours (with which are associated meanings that are themselves 'interactive' and 'social'). So, for Ahlemeyer and Ferrand and Snijders alike the fundamental components of the interaction are communications between the sexual partners.

Rather than pitting the concepts of individual-oriented and interaction-oriented perspectives against each other, or ignoring one or the other, another avenue is recasting them so they complement each other. Ingham and van Zessen tackle this key idea and demonstrate that individual characteristics and the elements of the context 'become salient only during the interaction itself', which means, *a contrario*, that many individual characteristics have no importance for the interaction itself.

To summarize the authors' positions, the individual is seen as a social actor characterized by a set of interactive behaviours that Max Weber (1978) would call social – they are performed in response to other actors. The social actor does not exist outside the interactions of which he is a part. The interaction is as real as the partners who are involved in it. Far from denying the reality of the individual, giving the interaction a more central position in the various theories makes it possible to redefine the theories in such a way that they become better suited for understanding the individual's sexual behaviour.

The Actor and Structure

The question of the place of the actor's own behaviour in these models calls for further thought. In Chapter 4 we stress the relatively small place of the actancial explanation in certain interaction-oriented theoretical perspectives. The irony is that some of the models that are criticized in the following three chapters, expected usefulness theory, social learning theory, etc., rely at least partly on actancial explanations. In this type of explanation any phenomenon such as safer sex is considered to result from the behaviour of the actors who are part of a social context and whose actions are intentional.

It is interesting to note that major theoretical breakthroughs in sociology find connections between the actancial and structural dimensions of social phenomena that the bulk of traditional schools of thought have tended to consider opposites. In current sociology two ideas are generally accepted: 1) Individuals and groups are the actors in their own individual and collective scripts. They are the ones who erect the structures (institutions, values, norms, and rituals) around which their individual and collective lives are organized and create the social situations (socio-economic inequality, risky contexts, etc.) with which they must cope. They are not the passive toys of such structures, rather they change or renew them through their daily actions, decisions, inventions and social relationships. A large part of social science analysis ultimately boils down to deconstructing these collective entities and attaching probabilities to actions which are likely to be repeated. So, these structures merely appear to be objective. Everything occurs as if they existed in their own right (Gosselin, 1992; Van Campenhoudt, 1994). This is the actancial dimension of analysis in the social sciences. 2) However, these social structures impact these actors' later actions. They define a system of constraints (habits, internalized behaviour patterns, routine procedures, risks of punishment of greater or lesser severity, etc.) but still allow room for manoeuvre and deviant behaviour. The game is based only half on chance. Not all sexual behaviours are predetermined, but not every sexual behaviour is possible.

So, structures and actors complement each other. As we have seen, the theoretical perspectives presented in the first part of this book do not give these two analytical components in the social sciences equal weight, and they continue to have problems including them within their perspectives. Thus, Ferrand and Snijders envision the possibility of connecting social network theory and social interaction theory without truly having managed to do so. Given the difficulty of the task, they believe it is unwise to develop a comprehensive theory that would explain all AIDS risk-related sexual behaviour. Using Merton's idea of *middle range theories* (Merton, 1949) they are content with suggesting a thorough study of certain aspects of the problem, such as the influence of confidants on behaviour. In Ahlemeyer's approach, the communications between partners are the components of intimate systems. However, these communications are considered mainly with regard to their function of reproducing the system, not with regard to their ability to change the system or play an unforeseen game. The perspectives presented by Ludwig (see Chapter 2) and Bastard, *et al.* (see Chapter 3) are tied to relatively little-formalized material explanations that nevertheless take various structural and actancial dimensions of the interactions into account.

The challenge this section leaves us is to better conceptualize this mutual constitution of the structural and actancial dimensions of sexual behaviour *vis-à-vis* the risk of AIDS. Various theories from other fields of sociology and social psychology, which try to build systems of action, can open up a new avenue of investigation. Section III will make further contributions to this effort.

Another avenue is constantly to shuttle between the two approaches in a process where each approach is taken seriously but challenged by the other approaches and real-world experiences. Rather than trying to integrate the structural and actancial dimensions of social phenomena, this perspective, according to Franck (1994, p. 301), is the very essence of the dialectic explanation. Whatever the magnitude and quality of the efforts required to recompose the links between structure and actancial explanation, such a dialectic process, driven as much by recognition of the importance of speculation as by flawless scepticism of speculation, will always be indispensable. The three chapters that follow are linked by this scientific dialectic spirit. The authors' criticism of individual-oriented approaches is valuable in developing interactive-oriented perspectives.

References

BOUDON, R. and BOURRICAUD, F. (1982) *Dictionnaire critique de la sociologie*, Paris: PUF.

DEVILLÉ, P. (1994) 'Modélisation économique et explication causale', in FRANCK, R. (Ed.) *Faut-il chercher aux causes une raison? L'explication causale dans les sciences humaines*, Paris: Institut interdisciplinaire d'études épistémologiques.

FRANCK, R. (1994) *Faut-il chercher aux causes une raison? L'explication causale dans les sciences humaines*, Paris: Institut interdisciplinaire d'études épistémologiques.

GOSSELIN, G. (1992) *Une éthique des sciences sociales*, Paris: L'Harmattan.

LORIAUX, M. (1994) 'Des causes aux systèmes: La causalité en question', in FRANCK, R. *Faut-il chercher aux causes une raison? L'explication causale dans les sciences humaines*, Paris: Institut interdisciplinaire d'études épistémologiques.

MERTON, R.-K. (1949) *Social Theory and Social Structure*, Glencoe, NY: Free Press.

VAN CAMPENHOUDT, L. (1994) 'Recherche sociologique, éthique et politique', in *Variations sur l'éthique, hommage à Dabin, J.* Brussels: Publications des Facultés universitaires Saint-Louis.

WEBER, M. (1978) *Economy and Society: An Outline of Interpretative Sociology*, **2**, Berkeley, CA: University of California Press (*Wirtschaft und Gesellschaft*, 1922).

WUNSCH, G. (1994) 'L'analyse causale en démographie', in FRANCK, R. *Faut-il chercher aux causes une raison? L'explication causale dans les sciences humaines*, Paris: Institut interdisciplinaire d'études épistémologiques.

Chapter 5

From Individual Properties to Interactional Processes

Roger Ingham and Gertjan van Zessen

Introduction

Yeah, but you can't sort of say – can't have sex because of the risk of AIDS, can you? . . . They sort of say don't sleep around and have casual sex, but no-one cares, do they? Not a lot of people, young people especially. (16-year-old UK female)

Well, in cold blood and sitting here with my clothes on, it's very sensible and it's perfect and it's the thing you should do and obtain a full sexual history of your prospective partner, but you get in a dimly lighted room, wearing not quite so many clothes, with some-one you find attractive, you sort of feel a bit awkward. (19-year-old UK male)

Given the amounts of money, time and energy that are currently being in-vested in the area as a result of the AIDS epidemic, it is essential to have an adequate conceptual framework with which to approach the understanding of sexual behaviour. This is not only a necessity for science to advance, but is also urgently required if relevant and effective interventions to reduce the spread of HIV infection are to be implemented. The aim of this chapter is to share our concerns regarding the application of traditional, cognitive health and social behaviour models to the study of sexual activity.

Our target is the range of formal quantitatively based models that have been developed over the past twenty or so years to attempt to predict health-related behaviours. Starting with the Health Belief Model (Maiman and Becker, 1974; Rosenstock, 1974; Rosenstock, Stecher and Becker, 1988), various additions and adaptations have been made as different researchers have identified further components. Traditional social psychological models

(Ajzen, 1985; Ajzen and Fishbein, 1980; Rogers, 1983) have also been applied in the context of health-related behaviours and sexual activity. The underlying concept of individual rational decision-making that is implicit in these models has come under close scrutiny in recent years (Brown, DiClemente and Reynolds, 1991; Ingham, Woodcock and Stenner, 1992; Loewenstein and Furstenburg, 1991; Montgomery, *et al.*, 1989; Pollak and Moatti, 1989; van Zessen and Straver, 1991). We are not concerned in this chapter about the utility of these models as such, but rather their specific application and operationalization in the field of sexual behaviour.

Although the various models differ in respect of their specific constituent components, they are based on some common assumptions regarding the production of behaviour. It is these shared assumptions that lead to our disquiet and which we wish to address in this chapter. These assumptions can be summarized as follows:

- the formal models incorporate an individualistic bias that places insufficient attention on the relational and wider social and cultural contexts in which sexual activity takes place;
- they are built on an assumption of rationality in that they assume that there will be consistent and predictable relations between attitudes, cognitions, intentions and behaviour;
- they are static in that they attribute to individuals (and assume that these can be measured through questionnaires) certain fixed levels of properties such as knowledge, attitudes, perceived risk, perceived severity, and so on.

In discussing our disquiet regarding the applications of these models to the field of sexual behaviour we shall be drawing on research projects in which we have been separately involved in the UK and the Netherlands. Both projects have used qualitative research methods, in particular, in-depth interviews with young heterosexual people in which detailed aspects of their sexual activities were explored. The UK study involved 225 young people aged between 16 and 25 years (Ingham, *et al.*, 1991 and 1992), of which the first 125 have so far been thoroughly analysed. The Netherlands study involved 100 young people aged between 18 and 32 years who had been selected by the criterion of having had two or more partners during the previous two years (Rademakers *et al.*, 1991, 1992). All the interviews were tape-recorded and transcribed for detailed analysis and covered details of sexual histories, perceptions of risk and risk assessments, detailed accounts of recent sexual events and other related topics. Comparisons of both samples with larger surveys show that the samples are not atypical in terms of their sexual histories or activities.

Our research approach accords priority to the perspectives of the participants themselves, in contrast to model-driven research, in which the major dimensions of the particular theory are imposed upon the data. Our approach thereby allows the identification of broader and more personally relevant explanatory factors in terms of sexual activities in personal and social contexts. The core material of the Netherlands study comprises detailed accounts of two recent sexual interactions, one being the most recent occasion and the other being contrasting in some way, preferably in terms of safeness. The UK study involved rather younger people, collected details of sexual histories, and placed a particular focus on, amongst other things, the circumstances and events surrounding first-ever intercourse.

Analyses of this type of open-ended material examine the full range of responses and also involve the identification of recurrent themes in separate accounts. This latter exercise permits the formulation of themes and processes that are above or outside the level of individual awareness. As such, they are embedded within accounts, but individuals could not be expected to be able to articulate them. It should be stressed that the quotations included in this chapter are intended to be purely illustrative of themes, rather than arguments in themselves.

Although there are some interesting variations in the data collected in the two countries, we found consistent themes that ran through the accounts obtained. First, we consider some of the common components of the major models and point out some ways in which these do not adequately capture the reality of sexual interactions and decision-making processes. Next, we discuss ways in which the models fail to give adequate attention to the importance of social contexts and structural dynamics and raise some issues concerning the relationship (implicit in many of the models) between intentions and behaviour. Finally, we outline an alternative conceptualization of the field.

Components of Formal Models

In a review of the literature, King and Wright (1991) list and compare the constituent components of models concerned with the determinants of individual health behaviour. The 14 models contain a total of 22 separable components, but no single model contains more than seven of these. Nine components are found in no more than two models, indicating a degree of consensus about the major components. The following variables appear in these models: attitudes, behaviour, behavioural control, benefits, cost barriers, cues, demographics, efficacy, environment, informative influence, motivation, knowledge, normative influence, perceived efficacy, perceived severity, perceived susceptibility, psycho-social factors, reinforcement, risk, skills, solutions, and subjective norms.

We do not discuss individual models or all the various constituents, but limit ourselves to a brief discussion of key components. These are the perception of risk and the role of social factors. Perceived behavioural control (or self-efficacy) is discussed later. We shall not discuss knowledge as such, since there is empirical evidence that levels of knowledge and attitudes towards safer sex show little or no direct connection to behaviour (see also Pollak and Moatti, 1989). Although respondents often report uncertainty over the exact modes of transmission, due partly to conflicting and unclear information in campaigns and media, the essence of safe sex, i.e., using a condom to prevent AIDS, was understood by nearly 100 per cent of the participants in both the Netherlands and the UK studies.

Risk Perception

The role of risk perception in the models is often separated into awareness of risk, estimates of the magnitude of risk, personal susceptibility, and severity of the disease. All these perceptions are typically measured as levels of risk and as cognitions that are relatively stable over time and situations. Higher levels are assumed to predict more powerful behavioural intentions.

Interpretations of perceived levels of risk are extremely difficult when it is unknown by what mechanisms and in which contexts risk perception takes place. Abrams, *et al.*, (1990), for example, report that their respondents (aged between 16 and 19 years) believed that 50 per cent of their heterosexual peers would be HIV positive (and hence 'die of AIDS') within the next ten years, whereas their own personal level of risk was perceived as being very low. Such general perceptions of risk levels do not directly relate to the actual processes described by those respondents in relation to individual sexual interactions.

Further, the timing of risk perception is often ignored in studies that rely on questionnaire-derived and/or static data. In the Dutch study, 36 per cent of respondents reported that they typically assessed the risk after the event, when sexual contacts had already taken place. These *post hoc* reflections on risk therefore cannot be considered as simply contributing to a learning experience that leads to more timely risk perceptions in subsequent sexual encounters, but may represent a typical way of coping with risks. With other respondents, who made and checked their perceptions of risk before or during the actual contact, the estimation of risk appeared not so much a rational assessment of potential danger, but served a symbolic function. Thus, participants demonstrate that they are aware of the new discourse on responsibility and safety by engaging in a short mutual reflection on AIDS, without any direct behavioural consequences.

The same can be said for checking a partner's sexual past, which similarly often appears to serve a purely ritual purpose. The UK study showed that the interpretation of what was meant by *knowing* one's partner was highly ambiguous. Given that a major national campaign in the UK was based on the advice 'get to know your partner or use a condom' and the majority of respondents genuinely believed that they did indeed know their partners (through acquaintance at school, living in the same neighbourhood, etc.), a justification for not using a condom was readily available to them.

Analysis of detailed accounts of sexual encounters in the Dutch study shows that the perception or awareness of personal risk varies over time, in both magnitude and function. A stable estimate of risk over time was identified in approximately one-third of the respondents, who could be broken down further into two distinct sub-groups. Some had decided, as a general rule and irrespective of the partner, that AIDS was a risk that should be reckoned with even though the estimated magnitude of personal risk might be low. The others may have acknowledged similar levels of risk, but refused to allow this threat to affect their personal lives. The former group is illustrated by a Netherlands respondent who decided that she would use condoms irrespective of the impression her partners gave: 'There's always the question how well you can assess someone. You're always subjective. And if you wish someone to be healthy, you can convince yourself very easily that he is, can't you?' (30-year-old female). The latter is reflected by a young man in the UK sample who reported, 'I'm a chancer and I know I'm a chancer and I know I should really take care, you know, but – well, you know, with the AIDS thing, I know that I should use a condom' (25-year-old male).

The difference between these categories is not a difference in levels of perceived risk as such (which could be measured along a particular dimension), but reflects a different answer to the question whether one does or does not accept that AIDS has personal consequences. Other respondents were aware that AIDS constituted a risk but were completely unable to provide an estimate of the magnitude of such risk, whereas still others did not think in terms of risk at all. For yet another group, the estimates changed in magnitude or function in the course of sexual interactions.

Thus, not only is risk a concept that can be perceived, but the notion of risk can also be created (or inhibited) during the interactions themselves, in accordance with the perceived needs of the flow of the encounter, the presentation that one wishes to give, and so on. In such cases, however, the apparent function of raising the issue is often to minimize the threat, not to assess potential risk.

Social Dimensions

Many of the models under consideration incorporate a component that assesses the impact of a social dimension. Thus, for example, the Theories of Reasoned Action and Planned Behaviour use the concept of *subjective norm*, which is derived from the extent to which respondents believe that significant others would approve of a particular behaviour and the extent to which the respondents wish to comply with these referents. In practice, scores on these dimensions are multiplied to produce a score for the subjective norm.

Although there can be little doubt that social issues are important, the operationalization of these concepts does lead to some problems. One issue concerns who should be selected as the significant others. Schaalma, Kok and Peters (1993) use three groups, these being parents, peers and partners (based on earlier findings that identify these three others as being important in young people's lives). The perceived beliefs of these identified others are scored on a 7-point scale and weighted by the motivation to comply with them, which is referred to as the *injunctive norm*. Schmidt (1991) uses as significant others *people you know* and *current partner*. The outcomes that are measured are intention to use a condom *with a new partner* and *during sexual intercourse*. Whereas it is difficult to argue against the selection of these operational variables individually, they do, through the formal demands of the model, lead to a rather strange item. Thus, the young respondents are asked, 'Would your current partner approve of you using a condom with a new partner?' It is difficult to know how easy it would be for respondents to answer this!

More fundamentally, even though it cannot be denied that for many young people their parents are important, there is a difference between the extent and the domain of influence. In other words, this item is rather difficult for young people to answer in those cases where parents (or other significant others) might not approve (or even be aware) of their sexual activity. This is not to deny that friends and parents might well have an influence on general attitudes to sexuality, morals and values, but this is quite distinct from implying or assuming a direct effect on specific behavioural outcomes. The qualitative data collected in both the UK and the Netherlands indicate that very little, if any, attention is paid in actual sexual interactions to the perceived opinions of others apart from the partner him- or herself (and even this does not always apply). In the examples provided above, the operationalization of social impact on outcome behaviours as demanded by the models diminishes the importance of the social for the sake of individualistic conceptions regarding the generation of behaviour.

A related argument can be offered in relation to the use of the concepts of costs and benefits, which are central in the Health Belief Model. Similarly, studies using the Theory of Reasoned Action (and Planned Behaviour) incorporate such concepts as part of the attitude component. Many studies of sexual behaviour use attitudes to condoms as a predictor variable and (intended) condom use as an outcome variable (Richard and van der Pligt, 1991; Schaalma *et al.*, 1993; Schmidt, 1991). This emphasis on condom use is inevitable, given the demands of the models to focus on specific behaviours. However, by targeting just one specific attitude domain and one specific behaviour, they ignore a range of other issues. For example, qualitative work has demonstrated that there are many other ways to think about the notions of cost-benefit analyses over and above those relating to condom use and risk reduction. Thus, for example, Dutch research in the field of commercial sex has shown that decisions with regard to safe sex are embedded not so much within notions of health as within frameworks of professionalism (for the sex workers) and meaning structures regarding paying for sex (for the clients) (Vanwesenbeeck *et al.*, 1992).

In our own research on young people we have found that the terms in which people assess the costs and benefits of condom use relate to issues such as social reputations and include fears of being a poor sexual performer, concerns about appearing to be lacking in trust or, alternatively, an infection risk, or concern about being unduly influenced by health threats. The actual outcomes depend to a large extent on interactional dynamics rather than pre-existing attitudes. Situations create costs and benefits. For example,

> I planned to use them, and they were in my coat, only four metres away, but still, it's four metres. You are in someone's bed, and you want to do it and you are both in a certain state, and I was afraid for the moment that she would say 'ho, wait a minute' and that she suddenly would realize what the hell she was doing. (22-year-old Dutch male)

> She produced condoms from the glove compartment of her car . . . she just said, 'Do you know what these are for?', I said 'yes' and she said 'good – use it', so I thought 'right, fair enough' (17-year-old male).

In summary, analyses of accounts of real sexual interactions reveal that the notions of risk perception, social influences, costs and benefits as represented in the current applications of these formal models do not adequately reflect the complexity of the concepts that they are intended to measure.

Intentions and Behaviour

We have raised some doubts regarding the application of some of the concepts that are deemed to be predictors of behavioural intentions in formal models. We shall now turn to the issue of the supposed relation between behavioural intentions and behaviour itself. According to Fishbein, Middlestadt and Hitchcock (1991), 'Since intentions are the immediate determinants of behaviour, a change in the behavioural intentions should lead to a change in the corresponding behaviour' (p. 250). Consider, however, some data from a Dutch population survey (van Zessen and Sandfort, 1991). One thousand adults were asked, 'Suppose you have a new sex partner. Would you propose the use of condoms?' This intention was clearly expressed by 95 per cent of the respondents, and 75 per cent considered that this would be an 'easy task'. However, when asked how they would respond if the partner objected, 50 per cent of the men and 18 per cent of the women with the 'safer intention' reported that they would not insist. Thus, despite clear and specific intentions and an apparently high level of self-efficacy, the simple addition of an anticipated objection changes the picture dramatically.

An important issue is how such discrepancies should be regarded. In formal predictive models, such results might indicate a degree of self-deceit, false answers, overstatement of capabilities, or some such lack of consistency. However, an alternative way of considering such apparent inconsistencies is to accept that immediate situational factors play a considerably larger part in the determination of behaviour than many models allow for. In other words, people simply do not know what will happen in many situations, so the strong emphasis placed on behavioural intentions is inappropriate. This is a crucial issue in the evaluation of many models, since empirical applications almost inevitably place behavioural intention as the key outcome variable (for example, van der Velde and van der Pligt, 1991). In some cases, reported behaviour is used in the models, but this is nearly always reports of past behaviour; few studies use a prospective design, in which intentions at Time 1 are related to actual behaviour at Time 2. In fact, even in studies that have used past behaviour as a predictor of future intentions, disappointingly low levels of variance are explained (for example, Maticka-Tyndale, 1991).

It is common for authors who use formal models to end their articles with token gestures about the need to take more account of the possible role of, for example, emotions, situations and interactional dynamics (for example, Schaalma, *et al.*, 1993). However, it is not easy to anticipate how such processes could be fit into the structures of such models. A key distinction here is that between prediction and explanation. Whereas the models may be useful for the prediction of particular health-related behaviours in some domains, in our view it is the uncritical application of the models to the field of sexual behaviour that has caused the problem (the problem being that the levels of prediction are generally very low). Defining sexual activity as an individual health issue imposes certain sets of constructs onto the field, with the result that some crucial and essential elements of interactional processes are made invisible.

The problem of relating intentions to behaviour has been recognized in the development of formal models, as in the inclusion of the concept of self-efficacy in the Protection Motivation Theory (Rogers, 1983) and the Theory of Planned Behaviour (Ajzen, 1985), drawing on Bandura's earlier work on social learning (Bandura, 1982). Thus, the extent to which people feel they have the skills and motivation to be able to carry through their intentions is assessed and assumed to influence intentions directly as well as the relationship between intentions and behaviour. However, given the models' requirement that only specific, narrow behaviours be considered, the operationalization of this measure is often highly specific (for example, 'I feel I will be able to use condoms consistently with new partners').

Close examination of accounts of actual sexual encounters reveals that there are considerably more areas that influence condom-use outcomes. The Dutch study suggests the important role of verbal and non-verbal interaction and negotiation, not only about condom-use specifically, but, more importantly, over the more general aspects of the progression and meanings of sexual encounters. More precisely, not more than one-third of respondents demonstrated consistency between their risk perception, intentions and behaviour. For the majority, the use or non-use of condoms could only be understood in terms of the actual interaction processes. Furthermore, the data suggest that intentions do relate much more directly to behaviours once there is a strategy, a mental plan for how, where and when to introduce the possibility of condom-use or safer sex. What these data point to is the requirement for a more general notion of interactional competence in sexual contexts, and not just a specific focus on (anticipated) condom-use itself (see also Straver, 1986, 1991; van Zessen and Straver, 1991).

Thus, the functioning of self-efficacy would appear to be a rather complex issue that is hardly covered by current operationalizations in the modelling of condom-use. The role of the general interactional competence that self-efficacy refers to appears to be a much more decisive factor than the models assume, but it is ultimately in the interaction itself that behaviour is produced.

An alternative approach to the intention–behaviour relationship is to look more closely at the concept of rationality itself. Analysis of the UK transcripts has revealed a number of different ways in which young people consider the possibility of behaving in a consistent manner with regard to sexual activity (Ingham, 1993). A range of alternative positions was identified, including 1) rationality as known but personally unattainable; 2) rationality as not being at all feasible in sexual behaviour; and 3) rationality as defined by, and constrained by, discourses regarding heterosexual relationships. A fourth position, adopted by some, was the view that they could adopt a sensible (or rational) way of behaving if they wanted to, but that for the time being they had chosen not to ('you're young only once').

Wider Social Contexts

If there is an acknowledgement that greater attention needs to be paid to interactions and the meanings of sexuality, then the wider contexts in which these meanings of sexual conduct are defined and structured cannot be ignored. These include the direct context of the sexual relationship, which has been demonstrated to have a major impact on safe sex behaviour. For example, growing intimacy leads to lower recognition of potential risk and greater difficulty in persisting with condom-use, primarily because of conflicting messages about safe sex, on the one hand, and trust as prescribed within the dominant sexual scripts (Simon and Gagnon, 1987), on the other.

Sexuality is age, status and gender graded (Gagnon, 1989). Research using qualitative methods to explore the accounts of young women in the UK (Holland, *et al.*, 1991, 1992; Lees, 1986) and in Australia (Crawford, Kippax and Waldby (1993); Kippax, *et al.*, 1990) has revealed the crucial importance of an understanding of power relations. A consistent finding has pointed to the relative weakness of women in negotiating when and how they wish to engage in sexual activities. Such work draws heavily on discourse analysis, which suggests that the strength of discourse is that it defines what is accepted as normal or taken-for-granted behaviours for men and women. Discourses derive from and are reinforced by media images, conversation, fiction, textbooks, and many other sources.

Hollway (1984) identified three common discourses that govern heterosexual relationships, namely, the have–hold discourse, in which the aim of young women is to 'acquire' and hold on to a man for the purposes of protection and reproduction; the male sex drive discourse, in which males are assumed to have a need for a regular sexual outlet and it is the women's role to satisfy this need; and the permissive discourse, in which sexual activity is seen as pleasurable in itself and can be engaged in without implied commitment. Given the force and prevalence of such discourses, particular behaviours and potential actions become literally unthinkable.

This has at least two implications. First, since the ranges of conceivable responses that individuals perceive will vary across different groups (according to age, gender, subculture and nationality, for example), the very process of comparing individual scores on rating scales is called into question, since the scale anchors will have different implications and meanings. People only know what they know, and what sense can be made of comparing individuals who may be dealing in different ranges? If the idea of gender-based power relations is adopted, comparison of males' and females' answers on a seven-point scale of self-efficacy is problematic. Second, the whole issue that certain behaviours are under individual volitional control is strongly challenged.

An empirical illustration of the influence of the wider social context can be found in the work of Jones, *et al.* (1986), who attempted to account for the variation in rates of unwanted teenage pregnancies in different developed countries in terms of a series of indices of the cultures' openness regarding sexuality. Similarly, Straver (1986), in comparing Scandinavian and US youth, demonstrated the effects of the more prescriptive cultural scripts regarding sexuality in the US on the experience, competence and satisfaction of young people. What these studies illustrate is that the taken-for-granted assumptions regarding aspects of sexuality differ considerably between countries and almost certainly between subcultures within countries, according to gender, class, ethnicity, and other categories.

To sum up, it is insufficient simply to expand the models in order to

incorporate additional components like interactional dynamics; an appreciation of wider contexts is essential for the interpretation of individual responses.

Towards an Alternative Approach

We do not disagree with the salience of the existing model components that
we have commented upon and their role in the production of sexual outcomes. What we have tried to do, however, is to demonstrate some serious
problems in the ways in which they have been used in practice and to raise
questions about the fundamental assumption in these models that behaviour
in sexual contexts can be predicted on the basis of individual cognitions,
rational or not. We also objected to the minimization of the role of social
dimensions and to the absence of consideration of interactional processes.

On the basis of our research, we have identified a number of other factors
that, in our opinion, contribute to a fuller understanding and explanation of
sexual conduct. In this section we propose a preliminary outline of the ways
in which the concepts of the formal models and our own work can be integrated, based on a model formulated in the Dutch study (Rademakers, *et al.*,
1992).

The object of interest is not individual decision-making but the interaction
itself. From this core position, other aspects need to be considered in order
to arrive at a complete explanation of the course of events. Since individuals
enter interactions with all kinds of expectations, plans, desires, capacities and
histories, these need to be taken fully into account to the extent that they
affect the course of the interaction. We distinguish two layers of potential
influences. The selection of two layers is to some extent arbitrary and is based
on the degree of proximity of the factors to the events themselves. The
proposed structure is represented graphically in Figure 5.1.

In the centre (the arena) is the interaction. The focus of interest is any
event described as occurring during the interaction that has any relevance
whatsoever to the outcome of interest, which is defined as safer sex (including use of condoms). Thus, for example, a sudden fear of failing to achieve
or maintain an erection may be a direct reason for not wishing to risk using
condoms. A further example comes from the UK data, in which interactional
events clearly played an important part. The circumstances of first-ever intercourse are described by a 17-year-old woman with a partner in his thirties:

> He came over and kissed me and I thought 'Oh, I can't do this', you
> know, and he was going 'Why not? why not? It doesn't matter.' The
> old line 'you can't get pregnant first time'. [Interviewer: Is that what
> he said?] Yes, which I . . . I didn't believe him, but still went ahead
> and did it without any sort of . . . I remember thinking, 'I'm stupid',

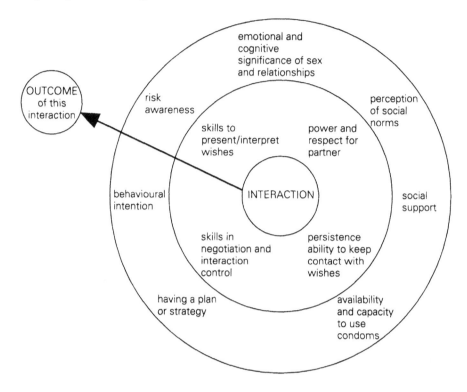

Figure 5.1 A preliminary dynamic model of sexual interaction (From: Rademakers, *et al.*, 1992.)

but still being that stupid, if you know what I mean. (17-year-old female)

The inner layer contains factors that are directly relevant for interactional functioning (competence):

- skills in presenting own and interpreting other's wishes;
- skills in negotiation and interactional control;
- power and respect for the partner;
- persistence or the ability to keep in contact with one's original wishes.

The outer layer contains factors that are relevant for, but not directly related to any one specific interaction:

- risk awareness;
- behavioural intention (which can be specific or general);
- having a plan and/or concrete strategy(ies);
- availability of and capacity to use condoms;

- perception of social norms;
- (perception of) social support;
- emotional and cognitive significance of sexual contacts and relationships.

Characteristic of this approach is not only that interaction is the central event, but also that individual and situational factors become salient only during the interaction itself. An intention to use condoms, a tendency to control the situation, a wish for a dominant position – all these factors have no salience outside the course of interaction, where the partners together create the outcome, even if one of them adopts a passive role.

Factors in either layer may be made redundant depending on the influence and impact of the factors nearer the core. An extreme example is rape, where all individual factors (for the victim) are overruled. Likewise, the 'intention to use condoms' (outer layer) may be overruled either by factors from the inner layer (such as a fear of raising the topic) or by something that occurs during the course of the interaction. The model presented needs to be expanded through the addition of time dimensions. It is important to gain a greater understanding of the ways in which different factors become more or less salient as a particular relationship develops (for example, a number of authors have pointed to the difficulties involved in continuing to insist on condom-use as a relationship becomes more firmly established, since to do so implies a lack of trust that is antithetical to increasing intimacy – see, for example, Holland, *et al.*, 1991, 1992).

The other dimension would be concerned with the development of individuals in terms of sexual careers and the processes by (or through) which individuals acquire a range of competencies, alternative sexual scripts, and so on. We suggest that the relationships between and the salience of the components identified in Figure 5.1 will vary as individuals experience new relationships and interactions. Mapping the ways in which individuals develop competence is essential to enable the design of suitable and appropriate interventions. We do note the start made in the interesting analyses by Schaalma, *et al.* (1993), which investigate the impact of the level of sexual experience of individuals on the relationships between the components of the Theories of Reasoned Action and Self-efficacy. We would, however, argue that such an approach would benefit from work that adopted a longitudinal approach and was also less restrained by the formal demands of the models used.

It is important to stress that the intention behind the model proposed here differs considerably from that more traditionally assumed in health-related behaviour studies. The essence of the distinction is that between prediction and explanation. We believe that, at this stage in the development of our understanding of sexual behaviour amongst young people, greater effort must be directed towards explanation than has hitherto been the case. This involves adopting a wider range of methods and being less constrained by the dimensions of existing models that have been developed to explore other areas of interest.

Conclusions

We started by drawing attention to some of the fundamental assumptions of the more dominant approaches to understanding health-related behaviour and our disquiet regarding their relevance to the study of sexual behaviour. These assumptions relate to the individualistic bias, the application of the concept of rationality, and the ways in which static properties are assumed to not only exist, but also be measurable. We have attempted to show, using data from studies conducted independently in two countries, that such basic notions do not, to any large extent, assist in understanding and explaining the events that occur in sexual encounters amongst young people. Greater attention needs to be paid to dynamic interactional processes.

The alternative approach presented here requires a great deal of research to explore its potential. We propose that a shift in emphasis is needed, away from the tendency of continual adjustment of models by adding more *boxes* in an effort to account for higher levels of variance and towards a focus on understanding. Given the importance of obtaining information about actual events and the ways in which people make sense of them, we suggest that qualitative methods, including individual account collection, group discussions, role-plays, and others, are essential for this task. It may be that it will be possible in the long run to capture some of these dynamic processes in quantitative terms. We are not against quantitative research as such – we see an important role for the continued monitoring of patterns of sexual activity or prevalences of beliefs to assess intervention effectiveness, for example, and for epidemiological purposes. It is the interpretation of such data, relying on models of individual and rational decision-making, that we wish to challenge.

Most of the recent research into sexuality is motivated by the urgent problem of AIDS. Research has been focused almost entirely on health and prediction, and less on understanding the role of sexual interactions. Gagnon (1988), in noting this problem, formulates two consequences. The first consequence of this concern with disease is 'that what is interesting about sex is what the disease makes interesting' (p. 600). The selection of the questions that are posed is generated by a concern for transmission or other disease- and health-related questions. A stronger consequence is:

> that sex itself can become confused with disease and being sexual in various ways becomes treated as an illness or as evidence of illness . . .
> Even within the constraints of a concern for AIDS, a narrow view of sexual behavior may be effective if all that we are concerned with is social book-keeping and epidemiological modelling, but it will be inadequate to the task of *understanding behavior in a way that results in behavior change*. Sexual conduct is embedded in culture and in social

relations – as we begin to deal with this dimension . . . we will need
to know a great deal more about the why. (Gagnon, 1989, p. 500)

References

ABRAMS, D., ABRAHAM, C., SPEARS, R. and MARKS, D. (1990) 'AIDS invulnerability:
relationships, sexual behaviour and attitudes among 16–19 year olds', in AGGLETON,
P., DAVIES, P. and HART, G. (Eds) *AIDS: Individual, Cultural and Policy Dimensions*,
Basingstoke: Falmer Press, pp. 35–52.

AJZEN, I. (1985) 'From intentions to actions: A theory of planned behavior', in KUHL,
J. and BECKMANN, J. (Eds) *Action Control: From Cognitions to Behavior*, pp. 11–39,
Berlin: Springer Verlag.

AJZEN, I. and FISHBEIN, M. (1980) *Understanding Attitudes and Predicting Social Behavior*,
Englewood Cliffs, NJ: Prentice-Hall.

BANDURA, A. (1982) 'Self-efficacy mechanism in human agency', *American Psychologist*,
37, pp. 122–47.

BROWN, L.K., DiCLEMENTE, R.J. and REYNOLDS, L.A. (1991) 'HIV prevention for
adolescents: Utility of the health belief model', *AIDS Education and Prevention*, **3**
(1), pp. 50–9.

CRAWFORD, J., KIPPAX, S. and WALDBY, C. (1993) 'Heterosexual men and Safe Sex
Practices', *Sociology of Health and Illness*, **15** (2), pp. 246–56.

FISHBEIN, M., MIDDLESTADT, S.E. and HITCHCOCK, P.J. (1991) 'Using information to
change sexually transmitted disease-related behaviors: An analysis based on the
theory of reasoned action', in WASSERHEIT, J.N., ARAL, S.O. and HOLMES, K.K.
(Eds) *Research Issues in Human Behavior and STDs in the AIDS Era*, Washington,
DC: ASM, pp. 243–57.

GAGNON, J.H. (1988) 'Sex research and sexual conduct in the era of AIDS', *JAIDS*, 1,
pp. 593–601.

HOLLAND, J., RAMAZANOGLU, C., SCOTT, S., SHARPE, S. and THOMSON, R. (1991)
'Between embarrassment and trust: Young women and the diversity of condom
use', in AGGLETON, P., HART, G. and DAVIES, P. (Eds) *AIDS: Responses, Interventions and Care*, London: Falmer Press, pp. 127–48.

HOLLAND, J., RAMAZANOGLU, C., SCOTT, S., SHARPE, S. and THOMSON, R. (1992) 'Pressure, resistance, empowerment: Young women and the negotiation of condom-
use', in AGGLETON, P., DAVIES, P. and HART, G. (Eds) *AIDS: Rights, Risk and Reason*,
London: Falmer Press, pp. 142–62.

HOLLWAY, W. (1984) 'Gender difference and the production of subjectivity', in
HENRIQUES, J., HOLLWAY, W., URWIN, C., VENN, C. and WALKERDINE, V. (Eds)
Changing the Subject; Psychology, Social Regulation and Subjectivity, London: Methuen,
pp. 227–63.

INGHAM, R. (1993) 'Some speculations on the concept of rationality', in ALBRECHT,
G. (Ed.) *Advances in Medical Sociology*, Vol IV: *A Reconsideration of Models of Health
Behavior Change*, Greenwich, CT: JAI Press, pp. 89–111.

INGHAM, R., WOODCOCK, A. and STENNER, K. (1991) 'Getting to know you . . . young people's knowledge of their partners at first intercourse', *Journal of Community and Applied Social Psychology*, 1 (2), pp. 117–32.

INGHAM, R., WOODCOCK, A. and STENNER, K. (1992) 'The limitations of rational decision making models as applied to young people's sexual behaviour', in AGGLETON, P., DAVIES, P. and HART, G. (Eds) *AIDS: Rights, Risk and Reason*, London: Falmer Press, pp. 163–73.

JONES, E.F., FORREST, J.D., GOLMAN, N., HENSHAW, S., LINCOLN, R., ROSOFF, J., WESTOFF, C. and WULF, D. (1986) *Teenage Pregnancy in Industrialized Countries*, New Haven, CT: Yale University Press.

KING, A.J.C. and WRIGHT, N.P. (1991) 'The design of HIV risk-reduction interventions: An analysis of barriers and facilitators', Report produced for the Global Programme on AIDS (YGP/IDS), World Health Organization, Geneva, by the Social Program Evaluation Group, Queens University, Kingston, Ontario.

KIPPAX, S., CRAWFORD, J., WALDBY, C. and BENTON, P. (1990) 'Women negotiating heterosex: Implications for AIDS prevention', *Women's Studies International Forum*, 13 (16), pp. 533–42.

LEES, S. (1986) *Losing Out: Sexuality and Adolescent Girls*, London: Hutchinson.

LOEWENSTEIN, G. and FURSTENBERG, F. (1991) 'Is teenage sexual behaviour rational?', *Journal of Applied Social Psychology*, 21, pp. 957–86.

MAIMAN, L.A. and BECKER, M.H. (1974) 'The Health Belief Model: Origins and correlates in psychological theory', in BECKER, M.H. (Ed.) *The Health Belief Model and Personal Health Behavior*, Thorofare, NJ: C.B. Slack, Inc.

MATICKA-TYNDALE, E. (1991) 'Sexual scripts and AIDS prevention: Variations in adherence to safer-sex guidelines by heterosexual adolescents', *Journal of Sex Research*, 28, pp. 45–66.

MONTGOMERY, S.B., JOSEPH, J.G., BECKER, M.H., OSTROW, D.G., KESSLER, R.C. and KIRSCHT, J.P. (1989) 'The Health Belief Model in understanding compliance with preventative recommendations for AIDS: How useful?', *AIDS Education and Prevention*, 1, pp. 303–23.

POLLAK, M. and MOATTI, J-P. (1989) 'HIV risk perception and determinants of sexual behaviour', in HUBERT, M. (Ed.) *Sexual Behaviour and Risks of HIV Infection*, Brussels: Facultes universitaires Saint-Louis, pp. 17–44.

RADEMAKERS, J., LUIJKX, J.B., VAN ZESSEN, G., ZIJLMANS, W., STRAVER, C. and VAN DER RIJT, G. (1991) 'Interactional aspects in the production of heterosexual behaviour', presentation at The 17th Annual IASR Meeting, Barrie, Ontario Canada, 6–10 Aug.

RADEMAKERS, J., LUIJKX, J.B., VAN ZESSEN, G., ZIJLMANS, W., STRAVER, C. and VAN DER RIJT, G. (1992) *AIDS-preventie in heteroseksuele contacten*, Amsterdam: Swets & Zeitlinger.

RICHARD, R. and VAN DER PLIGT, J. (1991) 'Factors affecting condom-use among adolescents', *Journal of Community and Applied Social Psychology*, 1 (2), pp. 105–16.

ROGERS, R.W. (1983) 'Cognitive and physiological processes in fear appeals and attitude change: A theory of protection motivation', in CACIOPPO, J.R. and PETTY, R.E. (Eds) *Social Psychology: A Sourcebook*, New York: Guildford Press, pp. 153–76.

ROSENSTOCK, I.M. (1974) 'Historical origins of the Health Belief Model', *Health Education Monographs*, **2**, pp. 328–35.

ROSENSTOCK, I.M., STRECHER, V.J. and BECKER, M.H. (1988) 'Social Learning Theory and the Health Belief Model', *Health Education Quarterly*, **15**, pp. 175–83.

SCHAALMA, H., KOK, G. and PETERS, L. (1993) 'Determinants of consistent condom use by adolescents: The impact of experience with sexual intercourse', *Health Education Research: Theory and Practice*, **8** (2), pp. 255–69.

SCHMIDT, P. (1991) 'Perspectives from the Theory of Planned Behaviour for explaining sexual behavior and evaluating prevention strategies', presentation at Workshop, EC Concerted Action on Sexual Behaviour and risks of HIV-infection, Sesimbra, Portugal, 31 Oct.–2 Nov.

SIMON, W. and GAGNON, J.H. (1987) 'Sexual scripts, permanence and change', *Archives of Sexual Behavior*, **15**, pp. 97–120.

STRAVER, C. (1986) 'De trapsgewijze interactie-carriere', in RADEMAKERS, J. and STRAVER, C. (Eds) *Van Fascinatie naar Relatie*, Zeist: NISSO, pp. 1–127.

STRAVER, C. (1991) 'Interactional processes in the construction of sexual contacts: A theoretical outline', presentation at The 17th Annual IASR Meeting, Barrie, Ontario Canada, Aug. 6–10.

VAN DER VELDE, F.W. AND VAN DER PLIGT, J. (1991) 'AIDS-related health behavior: Coping, protection motivation, and previous behavior', *Journal of Behavioral Medicine*, **14**, pp. 429–51.

VANWESENBEECK, I., DE GRAAF, R., VAN ZESSEN, G., STRAVER, C. and VISSER, J. (1992) 'Factors influencing safe sex in heterosexual prostitution', presentation at The VIII International Conference on AIDS/III STD World Congress, Amsterdam, 19–24 July.

VAN ZESSEN, G. and SANDFORT, T. (1991) *Seksualiteit in Nederland*, Amsterdam: Swets & Zeitlinger.

VAN ZESSEN, G. and STRAVER, C. (1991) 'Towards an alternative model of sexual behaviour', presentation at Workshop EC Concerted Action on Sexual Behaviour and risks of HIV-infection, Sesimbra, Portugal, 31 Oct.–2 Nov.

Chapter 6

Understanding HIV Risk-related Behaviour: A Critical Overview of Current Models

Jean-Paul Moatti, Dominique Hausser and Demosthenes Agrafiotis

Since the World Health Organization set up its Global Programme on AIDS, those in charge of this programme, in agreement with most public health officials, have stressed that information and education are the cornerstones of HIV control, since encouraging responsible behaviour by providing full information on the subject can be an effective means of preventing the transmission of the virus (Mann and Kay, 1988). Early social sciences research on AIDS, which consisted of surveys on the knowledge, attitudes, beliefs and practices of various sections of the population with regard to this epidemic (KABP studies), replicated findings obtained in other health education areas, such as prevention of smoking, prevention of cardiovascular diseases, or promotion of birth-control. Apart from some methodological and even epistemological difficulties in defining the concepts of beliefs and attitudes (Downie, Fife and Tannahill, 1991; Homar and Kahle, 1988), it seems to be fairly easy to correlate knowledge and beliefs with individual and collective attitudes towards the disease. However, the links often become more tenuous, not to say completely illogical, when one analyses reported behaviour on the basis of people's statements or actual behaviour based on direct observation.

Although risks awareness is obviously a prerequisite for prevention, improving the information available about the risks does not suffice to change people's behaviour in order to reduce their exposure to the risks of HIV infection (Moatti and Serrand, 1989). This initial series of investigations was thus followed by a second series designed to analyse the determinants underlying individual risk behaviours as regards the sexual transmission of HIV, borrowing some traditional models for individual behavioural change from the field of social psychology. These studies, which were mainly by North

American authors, revealed a number of behavioural factors associated with risk exposure that it was hoped might be useful for preventive purposes (Coates, 1990). These behavioural models seem, however, to be of little explanatory or predictive use. As we propose to show below, most of their work can be understood and critically reviewed in the framework of expected utility theory, a classic theory in the field of micro-economics dealing with individual reasoning in response to risk and uncertainty. We conclude by suggesting some possible lines of future research which converge with those presented elsewhere in this book. Our aim is to adopt a broader outlook than that underlying the mechanistic and reductive rationale on which the models mentioned above have been based. We feel there is a need for an analytical approach that attaches greater importance to the context surrounding HIV risk exposure and the dynamic time factors involved, particularly those relating to each individual's background and experience.

Knowledge–Beliefs–Attitudes–Behaviour: The Impossible Chain

Numerous before-and-after studies on the effects of advertising and educational campaigns for preventing HIV infection have shown that such actions improve people's knowledge about the disease and their awareness of the risks. They also help to build up attitudes reflecting solidarity with and empathy for those who have already contracted the disease. It has been practically impossible, however, to prove with any certainty that measures of this kind significantly affect behaviour, including the resolutions people admit to making about their own future behaviour (Stoller and Rutherford, 1989). It has likewise been reported that although press and media campaigns organized by public authorities can sometimes create a context that is favourable to prevention (developing HIV-risk awareness in the population, removing the mystique from the condom's public image, or re-adjusting social norms so as to promote solidarity with AIDS sufferers), it is quite impossible to prove that campaigns of this kind have ever been directly responsible for any real changes in behaviour patterns (De Vroome, *et al.*, 1990; Hausser, *et al.*, 1987, 1988, 1991; Lehmann, *et al.*, 1987; Moatti, *et al.*, 1992).

Many KABP (knowledge–attitudes–beliefs–practices) studies, which have been carried out in various countries on various sectors of the population, have shown the existence of significant statistical relationships between beliefs about the modes of HIV transmission and social attitudes towards HIV carriers. In the joint KABP–ACSF (Analyse des Comportements Sexuals en France) Sexual behaviour Survey study carried out in February and March 1992 on a sample of the French population between the ages of 18 and 69 years (Moatti *et al.*, 1992) the following parameters of measurement were

constructed: a *knowledge* score based on questions about scientifically established modes of HIV transmission; a *sensitivity to risk of HIV transmission* score
involving theoretically possible modes of HIV transmission that have practically
no epidemiological correlates, such as dental care; and a score on *tolerance*
based on a questionnaire about everyday attitudes towards HIV carriers using
the social interaction scale devised by Kelly, *et al.*, 1987. Several of these
parameters were significantly related (p < 0.001). Being properly informed
about the modes of transmission enhanced people's tolerance. Conversely,
the more people seemed to worry about the risk of infection due to either
uncertainty or a lack of explicit information, i.e., the more they tended to
believe that risks could be run in activities which can theoretically lead to
contracting AIDS in very rare cases, the less open-minded their attitudes were
towards AIDS sufferers.

The results of the KABP studies carried out in Switzerland since 1986 to
assess the outcome of the prevention campaigns launched by the public authorities (Table 6.1) likewise show how difficult it can be for researchers or
policymakers to differentiate between ideas that have been formed because
some risks are theoretically possible (although there exists no epidemiological
evidence). Those that are based on accurate scientific assessments, and traditional lay notions that may run contrary to the scientific evidence available

Table 6.1 Beliefs in HIV transmission (Switzerland)

Possible transmission	1986 Switzerland[1] age 20–69 n = 986	1987 Switzerland[2] age 17–30 n = 1211	1988 Tessino[3] recruits n = 1480	1990 Switzerland[4] age 20–70 n = 1007
	per cent	per cent	per cent	per cent
Sex	88	99	99	98
Shared syringes	23	95	98	99
Transfusion in Switzerland	54	43	47	56
Kissing/saliva	26	–	–	16
Kissing	–	–	5	–
Dentist	–	–	23	21
Handshake	32	–	1	1

[1] HAUSSER D., LEHMANN, P., GUTZWILLER, F. *et al.* (1986) *Evaluation de l'impact
de la brochure tous ménages d'information sur le SIDA distribuée par l'OFSP IUMSP,*
Lausanne (Cah Rech Doc IUMSP 7).
[2] HAUSSER D., LEHMANN, P., DUBOIS-ARBER, F. (1987) *Evaluation des campagnes de
prévention contre le SIDA en Suisse sur mandat de l'Office fédéral de la santé publique,
rapport de synthèse.* IUMSP, Lausanne (Cah Rech Doc IUMSP 23).
[3] DUBOIS-ARBER, F., LEHMANN, P., HAUSSER, D. *et al.* (1989) *Evaluation des
campagnes de prévention du SIDA en Suisse.* Deuxième rapport de synthèse 1988.
IUMSP, Lausanne (Cah Rech Doc IUMSP 39).
[4] VILLARET, M., DOMENIGHETTI, G. (1990) *Connaissances, opinions et préoccupations
de la population suisse et tessinoise vis-à-vis de l'épidémie de Sida.* Département des
affaires sociales. Service de la santé publique, Bellinzona.

at any particular time when interpreting beliefs about some of the modes of transmission.

The study carried out in 1989 in Athens (Agrafiotis *et al.*, 1989) again showed the existence of a gap between what the study population knew in general about the modes of HIV transmission and the difficulty the respondents had in assessing the respective risks involved in various situations. All around the world, at least as far as can be judged from the studies carried out in France, Switzerland, Greece, Togo and Mauritius (Agrafiotis, *et al.*, 1991), it has been observed that the higher the respondents' level of education, the less likely they are to believe in the scientifically disproved idea that AIDS can be transmitted simply by casual contact. The distinctions that can be made between people's beliefs based on their level of education are much less clear-cut, however, when it comes to modes of transmission, where there is still room for discussion as to the amount of risk involved.

In fact, questionnaires about the modes of HIV transmission should not be analysed in terms of right and wrong learning of the information available, but rather in terms of beliefs, which result from a complex alchemy between the availability of the relevant information and the way in which this information is interpreted in the wider context of the social images associated with the disease. For example, among the respondents participating in the 1992 French study, a higher percentage of those with lower than school-leaving certificate qualifications (41 per cent) than the percentage of college and university graduates (32 per cent) (p < 0.01) were able to produce the correct response that HIV can be transmitted from mother to child through breast-feeding (a fact recently established in the scientific press). This statistical difference obviously cannot be explained by saying that the respondents from the lower socio-economic strata were more assiduous readers of the *New England Journal of Medicine* than graduates of higher education. The authors of some qualitative studies have suggested that the idea of possible contamination by any of the body fluids (blood, semen, breast-milk) is consistent with the traditional popular representations about the pathways of contagion (Jodelet, 1989); those with more education, on the other hand, had probably not yet heard about the scientific reports demonstrating the possibility of contamination by breast-feeding and therefore responded 'no' to this point so as to avoid being suspected of adopting an intolerant attitude. The outcome of most of these KABP studies, however, has been a disappointing lack of causal links between either popular beliefs or informed knowledge and attitudes on the one hand and people's reported behaviour on the other hand.

Not only social and behavioural scientists, but also those in charge of prevention itself keep coming up against *the apparently paradoxical fact that individuals will go on exposing themselves to HIV risks even when they are perfectly aware of the existence and the nature of these risks.* According to a rather naive opinion that is nonetheless quite widespread in health education, this fact might be taken to show that irresponsible behaviour of this kind must be attributable to uncontrollable or irrational impulses. It seems, however, that most social scientists have taken up the challenge and started looking for the factors and mechanisms responsible for this bewildering contradiction between what people know and what people do.

The Contributions and Limitations of Behavioural Research

Several studies, the most fruitful of which were on cohorts from the homosexual communities living in large North American cities where it was possible to combine medical follow-up with psychological, sociological and behavioural data, have made it possible to identify some of the variables that are systematically associated with a high probability that an individual will adopt HIV-related high-risk behaviours. Table 6.2, which is from a contribution by Coates, *et al.*, (1990), shows the variables found to affect risk behaviour significantly. These variables include socio-demographic and psychological factors as well as those relating to the social environment.

These findings incontestably assisted preventive interventions. In particular, they led to the so-called San Francisco model, which helped to bring about spectacular changes in the behaviour of the homosexual and bisexual communities in that city within a very short period of time. They also served as the basis of the practical recommendations that were used in this model intervention programme. The recommendations may nowadays seem rather obvious, but that was far from the case in the early days of the North American epidemic. It was actually quite an innovation to state that:

- Preventive measures designed to change individual behaviour must not only provide information but also have motivational effects (modifying individual risk perception, for example).
- Not only abstract knowledge, but also practical skills training is required.
- The norms of the community to which the target individuals belong have to be influenced in such a way as to favour prevention.
- The measures should be aimed not only at the individual (clinical practices, individual counselling), but also at captive groups (schools, workplaces, prisons, etc.), even whole communities (which need to be defined culturally and/or geographically).
- It is necessary to take into account individual and group cultural factors and constraints, and in doing so the health and social workers involved should avoid expressing any moral value judgments *a priori*.
- Peers and lay community leaders should be called upon to support preventive campaigns (Coates and Greenblatt, 1989).

This body of research nevertheless raises several questions, primarily due to the fact that the procedure used is nearly always the same, that is, a

Table 6.2 Variables associated with increased probability of HIV infection or AIDS-related high-risk behaviours in the international literature

Variable	Association
Cultural groups	Incidence of AIDS and high-risk behaviours is more frequent among ethnic minorities (blacks, hispanics)
Socio-economic status	Exposure to risk of HIV infection is more frequent in low socio-economic groups
Age	Older adolescents and younger adults are at greater risk of AIDS-related high-risk behaviours and seroconversion
Alcohol and drug use	Combining alcohol and drugs with sex has been found to be associated with high-risk sex and HIV infection
Knowledge of health guidelines	Knowledge may be related to change in the earlier stages of the epidemic
Health guidelines efficacy	The degree to which one believes information about methods for reducing risk is associated with reduction in high-risk behaviour
Perceived costs of prevention	Perception of loss of pleasure and difficulty in changing are related to continued high-risk behaviour
Perceived threat	Susceptibility to HIV infection predicts lower risk behaviour
Perceived self-efficacy	Belief that one has the skills necessary to reduce risk is associated with risk reduction
Peer support	Belief that peers support low-risk sex predicts low-risk sexual behaviour

Source: Adapted from Coates (1990)

regression analysis is performed on a dichotomous dependent variable – usually the use of condoms or having had at least one high-risk sexual experience (e.g., anal intercourse with no condom) within a given period of time. The result is taken to indicate whether or not a given factor actually has statistically significant effects (after making the appropriate adjustments to allow for the other factors) on the dependent variable of interest. One objection that can be made to relying systematically on an approach of this type is that it may give rise to what one might call a *disciplinary bias*. The tendency to focus consistently on variables of the same kind, although it certainly sheds interesting light on the attitudes and behaviour under investigation, might in fact mainly reflect the disciplinary competencies and preferences of the investigators in charge of these studies. Researchers' emphasis on their own field of competence is normal; but problems have occurred because most authors have rarely given any thought to whether explanations might exist at levels other than those of their favourite variables. What makes matters worse is that they have sometimes overestimated the explanatory powers of their own approaches and claimed theoretical generalizations which were clearly beyond the possibilities of one specific field of investigation. Thus, research has been carried out quite separately on the psychological factors (personality structure) liable to explain the variability of risk behaviour within a single population (Hornung, Helminger and Hattich, 1992) as well as on other psycho-social (such as *locus of control* or self perception of one's ability to control the course of events), sociological (importance of the supporting social network, effects of female economic dependence on the male partner, etc.), even situational aspects (differences in the degree of risk depending on the specific type of sexual intercourse) (Moatti, 1991; Davies, Weatherburn and Hickson, 1993).

The second objection which might be levelled at this approach is a basic epistemological objection, namely, that the approach yields overly mechanistic analyses. This is due to a lack of objective thinking about whether risk factors as diverse as biological variables, socio-demographic and psychological characteristics, social images, etc., can all be validly dealt with at the same level. Furthermore, this has led to dealing indiscriminately with the actual instruments used to measure these vastly different entities (responses to questionnaires, data collection on socio-demographic variables, attitude ratings, etc.). In short, there seems to be a great risk that after much tedious data collection and sophisticated statistical processing, all one obtains may be a largely tautological set of results where what is taken to be the explanatory factors is in fact nothing but another way of expressing the dependent variables the authors had set out to explain.

One example of an impasse of this kind is provided by a study of a cohort of more than 600 young people with humble social origins from several North American cities who were followed up regularly from adolescence to adulthood starting in 1984. The outcome of this study was the conclusion that the predictors of HIV risk-related behaviour in this population were a lack of social support, past traumatic experiences and a high personal risk awareness. In other words, being poor, in difficulty and fairly self-aware means that one is more exposed than the average person to the risk of HIV infection (Stiffman, *et al.*, 1991). Without wishing to engage in any heavy polemics on the subject, it seems quite safe to say that this example is far from being the only one of its kind in the international social science literature on AIDS. As long as the aim of this research was mainly to identify the factors involved in risk behaviour and to provide general guidelines for preventive purposes, the tautologies did not really matter. As we shall attempt to explain in the following section, this approach really becomes a blind-alley approach, however, if it is adopted as a basis when the research is to be carried a stage further and claims to shed light on the reasons for which behavioural changes do or do not occur by validating pre-existing psycho-social models empirically.

The Health Belief Model and its Derivatives: An Illusory Explanation

The urgency of the AIDS epidemic may have motivated many social scientists to recycle available theories for applications in this new empirical field very quickly. This clearly is not sufficient to justify taking the pre-existing psycho-social models available in the literature (such as the Health Belief Model or the Theory of Social Learning), each of which is based on a particular combination of factors liable to influence behaviour, and taking any of these models to be empirically valid on condition that regression analyses show that some, or all, of the factors included *a priori* in the model are statistically related to some indicator of risky behaviour (Rosenberg, *et al.*, 1992).

As far as HIV infection is concerned, the starting point of most empirical research of this kind, conducted with a view to developing an explanatory model for the determinants of risk behaviour, has been the Health Belief Model (HBM), which was initially put forward in a Finnish experiment on cardiovascular disease prevention (Becker, 1974; Janz and Becker, 1984). The model is based on the hypothesis that the probability of an individual's taking either preventive or therapeutic steps when faced with a specific health risk depends on a set of belief-related factors that are assumed to have complex multiplying effects on behaviour. These factors include perception of the individual's susceptibility to the disease, perception of the severity of the disease, perception of the benefits of preventive action, perception of the barriers to preventive behaviour, for example, the physical, economic and psychological costs involved, the perceived degree of certainty about the efficiency of preventive action, and demographic and psycho-sociological factors relating to this context, such as General Health Motivation.

The studies that have been designed along the lines of the HBM purportedly demonstrate that high individual perception of the risks and benefits likely to accrue from preventive action is a good predictor of behaviour change and that it is possible to modify the underlying perceptions and beliefs actively by reinforcing the images associated with the positive benefits of prevention (for example, by pointing out how carefree people who use condoms can feel) (Solamar and Dejong, 1986); by providing preventive behavioural skills training along with the information; and by increasing risk perception by broadcasting messages designed to trigger moderate levels of fear. Moreover, information that gives rise to fear is known to be most effective when the preventive behaviour being recommended will help to abate the anxieties or the fears evoked (Job, 1988).

Table 6.3 Opinions about condoms*

Per cent of respondents who totally or rather agreed with the following statements about condoms	Condom use in the last 12 months	
	No	Yes
	per cent	per cent
Limit one's sexual pleasure	60.7	45.2
Kill romanticism in relationship	57.3	46.2
Are in contradiction with real love	45.1	26.8
Create doubts about partner	42.6	27.1
Are only for youngsters	26.8	11.9
Are difficult to use	24.9	13.5
Should not be considered like ordinary consumer goods	28.2	19.1
Are shameful to buy	11.3	5.6
Are out-of-date	11.9	6.4

* Sexually active population over the last 12 months (n = 1716)
French KABP–ACSF 1992 Survey

One of the HBM's features that makes it so attractive is that many of these aspects tie in quite well with the empirical data collected in quantitative surveys on sexual behaviour. In the 1992 French KABP–ACSF study, the score obtained on reluctance to using condoms was based on the responses to nine questions about perception of the condom as an efficient means of HIV prevention and the difficulties involved. The highest ratings on this point were found for respondents who had never actually used a condom during sexual intercourse or who had not used one recently (Tables 6.3 and 6.4). A trivial example showing the importance often attached to the cost of taking preventive action is provided by the fact that the only objection to condoms raised most frequently by those who had used condoms over the past twelve months versus non-users (65 per cent to 61 per cent, $p < 0.05$) was that 'it would be easier to buy condoms if they were less expensive'.

These examples should make us think harder about the tautological aspects of these models. Health beliefs and perceptions can be taken *a posteriori* to be either causes or consequences of an individual's behaviour. Since people's statements about what beliefs lead to what behaviour and vice-versa are difficult to check, there seems to be quite a good likelihood that we are dealing with a vicious circle, where the beliefs serve just as much to rationalize behaviour after the event as to inspire it beforehand. For example, the non-condom users in Table 6.3 expressed a significant level of doubt about the effectiveness of this device as a means of prevention and expressed negative views about its social image and its effects on a couple's physical relationship and love for each other. Does this mean that the non-users actually refused to use condoms for these reasons, or were they simply rationalizing their

Table 6.4 Score on reluctance toward condoms according to personal experience with condom use*

	Respondent		
	Already used condom during lifetime	Never used condoms during lifetime	Used condoms during the last 12 months
No reluctance	per cent	per cent	per cent
(Score < 2)	21.2	9.8	30.6
Slight reluctance			
(Score = 2 or 3)	38.3	29.2	40.2
Moderate reluctance			
(Score = 4 or 5)	31.7	36.5	25.3
Strong reluctance			
(Score > 5)	8.8	24.5	3.8
Total Sample	100.0	100.0	100.0

* The score was obtained by counting 1 point for a positive answer (*totally* or *rather agree*) to each of the 9 items in Table 6.3. The closer the score was to 9, the more reluctant the respondent was to use condoms.

refusal *a posteriori*? It seems fair to say that much more give-and-take is needed between the results of quantitative surveys based on the use of questionnaires and other more in-depth studies using qualitative approaches than has been evident so far in the international literature if we are to overcome these interpretative dilemmas.

Another problem stems from the fact that the HBM school of thought has some difficulty taking into account the impact of collective and normative influences at work in the social environment on 'individual perceptions'. Risk perception indices and scales are particularly sensitive to this problem. A comparison of the answers given by the 18- to 69-year-old general French public in 1992 versus 1990 showed that fewer respondents felt they ran an above average (4 per cent in 1992 versus 3 per cent in 1990) or average (35 per cent and 25 per cent, respectively) risk of being infected by HIV. The evaluators of the Swiss prevention campaign (Dubois-Arber, *et al.*, 1989) noted as far back as 1988 that fear of the disease was following two contradictory tendencies: it was decreasing among the population at large, but judging from some increasing anxiety pointers, increasing perceptibly in the groups which had the most contact with the disease. Although by 1988 the panic reactions (about the threat to people themselves and their families) observed before the first large-scale Swiss information campaigns had disappeared, worry could often be detected at meetings about AIDS. Such concern was sometimes expressed indirectly in the form of requests for information and advice. Moreover, in some special situations, such as when a condom had failed to provide protection, and the results of a blood test were being awaited, people were sometimes extremely distressed.

The apparently contradictory decrease in the signs of fear and individuals' perceptions of the risk of infection which has occurred among the population at large as the epidemic takes on ever-increasing proportions has been observed not only in France but in other countries as well, including the United States, where 'the percentage of people perceiving themselves to be at a high risk of contracting AIDS has declined steadily since 1987' (Blendon, Donelan and Knox, 1992). Gauging the perceived risks seems, in fact, to involve a mixture of an awareness of the personal risk of HIV exposure and other more general subjective feelings about one's own state of health, along with a perception of the collective risk to which society as a whole (and hence the individual members of society) is exposed because of AIDS. This idea was suggested by the 1992 French KABP study, where individual perception of the risk of HIV infection was found to depend on people's general perceptions of their own state of health. According to this study, 24 per cent of those who felt their state of health to be not at all satisfactory thought they were more at risk than other people of being infected by the AIDS virus, whereas only 9 per cent of those who judged their state of health to be satisfactory were of this opinion. In the same way, the decrease in the risk perception level in the population as a whole seems to reflect a decrease in the diffuse social uneasiness which was felt about this unknown disease at the beginning, as well as a decrease in the gaps between subjective risk perception and the objective conditions of exposure to sexual transmission of the virus. In 1992, people's perceptions of their personal risk as being equal to or more than the average decreased, quite logically, with age (43 per cent were of this opinion among the 18- to 24-year-olds, 29 per cent among the 25- to 49-year-olds and 17 per cent among those aged 50 years and over). This feeling increased with the amount of sexual activity (56 per cent and 71 per cent among men and women having had two sexual partners or more during the foregoing year), and was also related to the degree of tolerance towards AIDS victims (59 per cent of those individuals who felt they were at average or more than average risk answered the five questions about tolerance towards HIV carriers in everyday life affirmatively, whereas only 50 per cent of those in the remainder of the sample answered these questions affirmatively). Finally, it is difficult in cross-sectional surveys of the population's risk perception to take into account the effects of past experience and those of previous contacts with the disease. For example, in one of our studies on pregnant women (Moatti *et al.*, 1990), individual perception of the risk of HIV infection was strongest, not among the women who had undergone a prenatal HIV screening test (on whom this test obviously had reassuring effects), but among those who had thought about the test but had not had the opportunity to take it.

Much debate has centred on what has been rather loosely referred to as the *relapse* phenomenon. This provides yet another example of how difficult

Table 6.5 Risk perception of AIDS and other health risks and diseases

	Assessment of relative importance among total mortality[1]			Individual fear of risk[2]		
	1990 Average /many	1992 Average /many	Level of Significance	1990 Average /high	1992 Average /high	Level of Significance
	per cent	per cent		per cent	per cent	
AIDS	69.5	77.9	N.S.	33.8	24.0	(*)
Road accidents	96.8	95.9	N.S.	75.8	74.1	N.S.
Cancer	95.8	96.7	N.S.	72.7	70.7	N.S.
Cardio-vascular disease	90.7	92.8	N.S.	59.8	52.2	(*)
Alcoholic diseases	87.9	88.0	N.S.	11.1	9.6	N.S.
Suicides	69.4	75.0	N.S.	12.4	7.2	N.S.
Occupational accidents	51.7	49.4	N.S.	26.0	19.4	(*)
Genetic diseases	39.4	47.0	N.S.	–	–	–
Hepatitis B	30.1	42.5	(*)	27.4	26.5	N.S.
STDs	26.2	42.1	(*)	15.3	14.1	N.S.

* $p < 0.01$ – chi-square test after adjustment for socio-demographic characteristics.
1 Respondent was asked to assess how many people died from each of these risks and diseases during the previous year in France: *a few, an average number,* or *many.*
2 Respondent was asked to express his individual fear of suffering or contracting each risk or disease: *quite small, average* or *high.*
Source: French KABP 1990, n = 916; French KABP-ACSF 1992, n = 1927.

it is to account for changes over time. The term relapse has been used in connection with a proportion of the North American homosexual and bisexual cohorts who, after giving up sexual practices involving HIV-exposure risks, have tended gradually to revert at least occasionally to their former habits (Ekstrand and Coates, 1990; Ekstrand, *et al.,* 1992). These so-called relapses cover several different phenomena, namely, the occasional return to high-risk practices in a specific context, persistent high-risk behaviour over a long period (particularly at the lower social levels), and giving up the use of condoms during a lasting relationship with a partner having a known serological status, which is a very different matter from relapsing as applied to somebody who falls back into habit-forming practices (drinking, drug abuse) after trying to give up the habit for a period of time.

The present alternative to the HBM seems to be the models based on social learning theory that have recently come to the forefront in the literature on AIDS risk behaviour. These models strive to identify the environmental conditions associated with behaviour and examine the various stages in any behavioural changes (Bandura, 1977; Leventhal, 1973; Leviton, 1989). In social learning theory behavioural change is taken to involve several phases, and individuals are assumed to envisage adopting protective measures and to search for information in the initial phase before definitely deciding to embark on the road to change. Great emphasis is placed on the idea that in this early stage individuals will take into consideration what they know about other people's experience. Like the HBM, these models certainly fit some of the empirical findings of behavioural surveys. For instance, the impression people had that their practices were based on the habits of those around them was the main variable found in some studies to be significantly related to a decrease in risk behaviour (Becker and Joseph, 1988). Declared use of condoms could often be statistically related to statements that the respondents felt they were in contact with HIV infection, since they personally knew at least one HIV carrier (Agrafiotis, *et al.*, 1989; Moatti, *et al.*, 1991). In the same way, analysis of the heterosexual respondents in the 1992 KABP-ACSF study who had engaged in sexual activity over the previous 12 months revealed a larger proportion of condom users among those who stated they were personally acquainted with a seropositive person (29 per cent) than in the rest of the sample (19 per cent). A similar pattern was observed when those who had the impression that their friends and acquaintances used condoms were compared with those who did not (35 per cent condom users versus 10 per cent condom users, respectively). However, exceptions to the general rule that acquaintance with the disease is associated with a higher probability of adopting protective measures are frequent, for many individual cases have been reported in which there seems to be no choice but to do without protection (statements by interviewees referring to the strength of people's feelings for their partner or to the unavailability of condoms at the appropriate moment) (Masur and Dubois-Arber, 1990).

The most highly developed social learning models have also included the notion of 'self-efficacy' (Bandura, 1977). The idea here is that individuals will assess their own ability to change their behaviour and update this self-assessment in the light of experience. Those who blame their failures on their own lack of ability will be more reticent about making a second attempt than those who feel that they did not try hard enough. The conclusions reached about personal experiences will depend not only on individual personality traits, but also on how people feel towards their own bodies and what they think about health and disease, i.e., attitudes that can be strongly influenced by the environment and prevailing social images.

Most of the criticism levied at the HBM also applies to the models of this second kind. First, both types of model tend to generate explanations in which too much reliance is placed on cognitive information processing. Second, they tend to consider that behaviour involving risk exposure is deviant or biased compared with an implied no risk or absolutely safe norm. In so doing they overlook some of the perfectly logical reasons for which risk-taking can be the outcome of an individual's rational decisions. The fact that

61 per cent of the men and 58 per cent of the women who participated in the French ACSF survey declared that choosing the right partners could be an efficient means of HIV protection, just as the majority of the Athenians questioned preferred this preventive strategy (Agrafiotis, *et al.*, 1989), will automatically be interpreted by these models as meaning that these individuals' idea of safety is illusory and liable to place them at risk. Perhaps what the respondents actually meant, however, when answering this question, was that, depending on what they could tell about a potential partner, they re-adjusted their assessment (consciously or otherwise) of the probability that the latter might have carried a prior risk of HIV or STD transmission (and that they therefore did not give the risk the same rating when they were with a close acquaintance as when they were with a stranger or a prostitute). In addition, it is quite likely that some of the respondents may have answered this question affirmatively mainly in order to show that they agreed with the norms and moral values prevailing in matters of sexuality.

The Expected Utility Model: A Disturbing Parallel with Behavioural Research?

Those who are not familiar with neo-classical micro-economics will no doubt be surprised to learn that links can easily be established between the psycho–sociological models of the kind we have been discussing and conventional economic models for risk and uncertainty behaviour (usually referred to as *expected utility theory*). As we propose to show below, the economic approach is furthermore based on a less reductive conception of individual rational decision-making than most of the health education models available for analysing behavioural determinants, although in the long run the expected utility models suffer from the same intrinsic limitations as all these other models due to their over-emphasis on *methodological individualism* in their approach to behaviours which involve social interactions. Therefore, our reference to the economic approach to individuals' rational choices does not claim to explain behaviours. Rather, it is used below as a critical tool to explore the limits of current psycho-social models.

If one compares even a highly over-simplified application of expected utility theory to decisions about condoms during one sexual encounter (Figure 6.1 and Appendix A) with the psycho-sociological models discussed above, it becomes obvious that the latter focus almost entirely on a single aspect, namely, the obstacles to rational individual choice due to either a lack of information or to a biased interpretation of the available information.

In the first place, subjective individual assessments of the probabilities p and q in Figure 6.1 are likely to differ from those of real-life probabilities, such as those established on the basis of the epidemiological data and by the

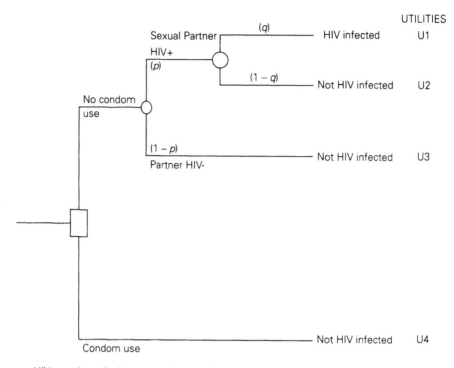

p = HIV prevalence in the community to which the sexual partner belongs
q = probability of HIV infection during one sexual encounter with an HIV positive sexual partner

Expected utilities
No condom use = $p[qU_1 + (1 - q)U_2] + (1 - p)(U_3)$
Condom use = U_4

Figure 6.1   Decision Tree about condom use during one sexual encounter

experts on AIDS, although there remains considerable uncertainty these days about the validity of these data. These differences can be decisive when individuals are not properly informed, especially if their perception and interpretation of the probabilities are biased in some way. Individuals' poor ability to make informed judgments consistent with the laws of probability has long been established in the field of experimental psychology. In the second place, it is possible that the relative values associated with the outcomes of the various branches of the decision tree (as to HIV infection versus non-infection) may have been reached on the basis of insufficient information. For example, the basic facts about what this infection means to an individual in terms of his future existence may have been glossed over. This possibility seems to be corroborated by the finding that subjective contact with the disease tends to be associated with a greater commitment to preventive behaviour and the fact that personal experience of close relatives or acquaintances suffering from the dermatological symptoms of Kaposi's sarcoma enhanced the motivation for prevention among homosexual cohorts (Becker and Joseph, 1988).

With regard to the first argument, Tversky and Kahneman (1974) have argued that individuals use a limited number of simplifying heuristic principles so as to keep only a reasonably small range of choices open and be able to adapt to the environment and that these heuristics often lead to serious errors in interpreting probabilistic information. These errors have been blamed on the *representativeness heuristic*, whereby probabilities are evaluated by similarity; the *availability heuristic*, whereby the frequency of events is judged on the basis of memory and imagination; and the *anchoring heuristic*, whereby a probability is judged in relation to an arbitrary starting point or anchor. Mechanisms of this kind have been found to operate to the full in uncertain situations where people's probability of survival rather than probability of monetary gains or losses is at stake (Fischhoff, *et al.*, 1981). As far as health risks are concerned, the mechanisms often result in biased probability interpretations due to either a fear of uncertainty, threshold reasoning (below a given probability threshold, an individual tends to assume that the personal risk to himself is negligible), sequential reasoning which leads to over-optimism (having escaped after an episode of risk exposure, such as remaining free of HIV infection after engaging in sexual intercourse with no precautions, tends to make people underestimate the risks associated with repeating the episode, even though the two probabilities are in fact independent), tendency towards over-confidence in one's own powers of judgment, and above all individual risk denial ('it can only happen to others') (Slovic, Fischhoff and Lictenstein, 1980).

The insistence on the barriers to acquiring probabilistic information and its accurate assessment should logically lead to the promotion of campaigns to correct the biases. Since we are dealing with a fatal transmissible disease, which raises what economists call the 'externality problem', i.e., one involving cross-effects between the risk to the individual and that to other individuals, there is a danger that coercive methods might become the last resort if it turns out that individuals will stubbornly resist all attempts to straighten out their information. Indeed, this step has already been crossed by those who claim that people put up psychological defences to avoid knowing about the risks to justify setting up repressive public health strategies, such as the creation of a judiciary system of supervision from which HIV carriers can be freed on parole (Archer, 1988); and by those who call for socially responsible reproductive behaviour to justify dissuading HIV-infected women from becoming pregnant and encouraging them to have an abortion if already pregnant (Arras, 1990; Krasinski, *et al.*, 1988).

The expected utility model draws attention to the fact that there exist other factors which can lead an individual to make a rational decision not to use preventive methods, even assuming that he has been fully informed about the risks. Individuals may have perfectly legitimate preferences for deciding whether or not to use condoms, including the latter alternative:

1   Even when people have been properly informed, the relative values (utilities) associated with the outcomes on each of the two decision branches can differ for many reasons. In particular, individuals may attach a relatively high value to the decision process itself (intermediate results), i.e., to elements such as the degree of pleasure to be derived, the simplicity of having sexual intercourse with or without a condom, and the psychological benefits resulting either from its use (such as freedom from anxiety) or from its non-use (such as pride in showing trust towards a partner with whom one is in love) (Cohen and Mooney, 1984).

2   Different individuals can have different preferences as regards risk-taking, i.e., they may react differently when faced with the same probability of risk. One of the main merits of the expected utility theory is that it has gone beyond the simple criterion of mathematical expectation by showing that people are not directly interested in the results of a lottery, but translate them into other terms, i.e., the utility of the results. When presented with the same lottery with the same probability of winning or losing, some individuals, the *risk-averse*, will be prepared to pay to avoid having to play, while the *risk-prone* would on the contrary demand compensation if they were prevented from playing. It has often been demonstrated that most people feel great risk aversion when confronted with lotteries where the gains and losses at stake are not money but health risks affecting life expectancy (Slovic, *et al.*, 1980). It has also been established however that this tendency becomes much less clear-cut when these probabilities are low, which is statistically true in the case of the present-day risk of HIV infection during heterosexual intercourse in Europe and North America (apart from some groups involving drug addicts) (Hellinger, 1989).

3   Another factor that can contribute to choosing non-protection and is likewise highly variable from one individual to another is a matter of inter-temporal preferences, which is evened out in traditional economic terms by applying a discounting rate. Thus, the current value of a health gain will fluctuate depending on the subjects' degree of preference for the present, just as the current value of one franc in ten year's time will be much higher with a low discount rate than with a high one (0.614 francs with a 5 per cent discount rate as against 0.322 francs with a 12 per cent rate). Now, in our illustration of decision-making about condom use one of the branches of the decision tree (non-infection) has immediate consequences, whereas the other branch (infection) will affect people's health only in the long term and may therefore be rated very differently depending on whether or not people attach more importance to the present than to the future.

4   Another point worth mentioning is that economic theory reminds us

that, generally speaking, the utility attached by an individual to extra gains decreases as his basic income increases (an additional franc is not greeted with the same degree of satisfaction by a millionaire as by a person living on meagre state allowances), whereas the utility of extra life expectancy gains tends to increase with the size of an individual's initial wealth (whether they are material ones or not). When drug abuse experts declare that interventions at the individual level are of little use if nothing is done about the social and economic conditions responsible for drug addiction, this amounts to saying that it is necessary to create an environment in which individuals will have an increased perceived utility of leading an addiction-free life in the future. The fact that the underprivileged lower classes tend to resist individual prevention much more than the middle and upper classes may likewise be attributable to socio-economic status-specific differences in the subjective value attached by individuals to a potential life expectancy gain.

Real-life and Rational Decision-making

The above reference to the expected utility model is not based on restrictive pre-conceptions of human rationality, which unfortunately are often shared by supporters of this economic approach. It is based rather on the alternative hypothesis that *real is rational* and that in a variety of socio-cultural conditions a variety of rationalities will emerge, the role of the social scientists being to try to understand these different rationalities even when they contradict dominant scientific practices and discourses.

In comparison with the predominant ideas and lines of research in the field of HIV prevention, the expected utility model at least deserves credit for pointing out that risk-taking results in many cases from perfectly rational and logical decisions, and that it has become necessary to do away with the over-simplifications such as assuming rational behaviour to equal zero-risk exposure. The only way of achieving an absolute zero-risk behaviour would indeed be to abstain completely from sexual intercourse, since one cannot ever be absolutely sure of a sexual partner's serological status. On the other hand, it would be an exaggeration to claim that models based on the expected utility theory framework enable us to understand the explanatory patterns underlying HIV-related risk behaviours and, conversely, the real mechanisms that lead an individual to pay the costs of adopting preventive behaviour.

The expected utility theory does not go any further than the psycho-sociological models, such as the HBM, in taking into account the obvious fact that the sexual transmission of HIV always involves intercourse between at least two individuals who belong to a complex network of social interactions.

Although at the theoretical level the approaches we have been criticizing were not in any way bound to overlook the socializing processes that all the individuals in a group undergo (Boudon, 1979), these individualistic methodologies often tend in practice to treat individuals as if they devised their own behavioural rules regardless of their memberships of various social groups and the specific contexts within which they interact. Their starting point remains 'the individual who, having preferences and being confronted with constraints, has to make choices' (Lindenberg, 1985). Even when norms, networks, environmental situations and dynamic processes such as learning and reflections are brought in as additional items on the individual's checklist in order to conceive 'new strategically rational actors' (Elster, 1979), social forces remain either restricted to those perceived or acknowledged by the individual or to an enumeration of additional constraints (Pescosolido, 1992).

In some ways, our criticism of all the models discussed in this chapter is in line with the distinction made by Augé and Herzlich (1984) in connection with disease in general. In the social sciences we have approaches where 'the medical definition of a disease is recognized as a biological reality imprinted on an individual body' and that view the social dimension of disease as consisting necessarily of 'the set of factors which affect the initial biological givens' (ibid.). We also have researchers who attempt to analyse health and disease (to which one might add attitudes towards risks) as if they were social constructs resulting from confrontations between the health professional's know-how and experience and the representations and practices of lay people. We believe that our criticism of current behavioural models is in line with this second approach and with recent trends both in the field of theoretical research on risk behaviour in general and among empirical studies dealing with AIDS.

Economic theory has developed a number of off-shoots in the form of studies attempting to transcend the expected utility theory assumptions' inherent limitations about rationality and to elucidate the true reasoning processes at work in the making of individual decisions. Loomes and Sugden (1982), for instance, have proposed a version of economic theory according to which the decisions taken by individuals *a priori* when faced with uncertainty are based not only on expected utility but also on the anticipation of negative feelings subjects will predictably have *a posteriori* if the final outcome is not what they expected. By dealing with the regret to be felt at the possible outcome of two compared courses of action, this approach has succeeded in eliminating the assumption of independence between probability and outcome that has been felt for a long time to be one of the main weaknesses of the classical expected utility models (Allais, 1953). To put it more simply, these authors assume that an individual will assess each possible decision in advance by wondering to what feelings of regret it will lead. Since choosing one form of behaviour means ruling out the other possibilities, an individual will feel either regret or satisfaction *a priori* when analysing each of the possibilities envisaged.

This idea looks as if it might be quite relevant to the question of HIV-risk prevention. When an individual makes one of several possible decisions, he compares the consequences and will theoretically opt for the decision commensurate with maximum expected utility, at the same time taking into account the potential associated regret. Deciding to take precautions during love-making may therefore lead to regret if avoiding disease by deciding to use condoms is compared with avoiding disease without bothering about prevention. In this case, combining the future regret with the expected utility can therefore lead to weakening the utility expected to accrue from preventive behaviour. Indeed, Tymstra (1989) has already observed that this regret model is in good agreement with the actual behaviour of patients faced with decisions as to whether extreme therapeutic solutions should be adopted (transplants, grafts, etc.). It might be worthwhile seriously considering the possibility of devising preventive slogans promoting the use of condoms where the stress is placed on the regret which will predictably result from not having used a condom during intercourse with a partner whose serological status is not known.

Times and Contexts

Most of the criticism that has been expressed in an attempt to improve the classical expected utility model has stressed the importance of the context surrounding risk exposure while at the same time attempting to adapt the model to a more dynamic picture of reality. From this point of view, these models have something in common with the latest social psychology research designed to eliminate the mechanistic and reductive tendencies that the previous models of the Health Belief Type suffered (Meter and Turner, 1992). A need for new models had arisen by this time, given the patterns of preventive practice, where, after a rapid increase, condom use has reached a plateau, which unfortunately does not mean that risk prevention has reached saturation, for adoption of safer sex has slowed (as in the case of the Swiss situation – Tables 6.6 and 6.7).

New lines of psycho-social research may develop from recent research on social identification theory, in which it has been attempted to extend the basic model of the social self as a mix of internalized group attitudes. Turner (1982) has suggested that the self-concept may be an organized cognitive structure which functions in a way which is both adaptive and situation specific. In a given situation, people may adopt any one of a number of possible selves, activating some salient aspects of their personal and social identities. Some behavioural situations (such as competitive situations and inter-group conflicts as well as affective or sexual relationships) engage people's sense of social identification with a particular group. Some other promising avenues

Table 6.6 Condom used with a new partner with whom a stable relationship was started during the last 12 months (Switzerland)

Age of respondents	Respondents who engaged in a stable relationship with a new partner	Condom use with this new partner
17–30 years	per cent	per cent
Oct. 88	20	40.8
89	15	52.2
90	17	55.2
91	14	56.7
92	14	66.0
31–45 years		
Oct. 89	4	56.3
90	3	54.3
91	4	52.1
92	4	68.0

Table 6.7 Systematic condom use with occasional sexual partners during the last six months

Age of respondents	17–20	21–25	26–30	31–35	36–40	41–45
	per cent	per cent	per cent	per cent	per cent	per cent
Jan. 87	16	6	3	–	–	–
Start of the Stop Aids campaign						
Oct. 87	20	19	5	–	–	–
88	51	28	26	–	–	–
89	53	45	48	30	18	16
90	73	37	42	43	30	31
91	58	51	45	44	33	32
92	69	61	50	47	51	61

of research are those involving a combination between quantitative surveys and qualitative social anthropology methods which have shown how the public develops a 'lay epidemiology' to 'accommodate official messages concerning behavioural risks within the important cultural fields of luck, fate and destiny' (Davison, *et al.*, 1991).

Another promising approach seems to be that of setting sociological research within its present-day historical context. Michel Pollak (1988) and Mitchell Cohen (1991) have proposed to take a historico–temporal viewpoint of this kind in their respective studies of the French homosexual community and homosexual communities of San Francisco and Amsterdam, arguing that such a viewpoint can demonstrate specific groups of factors as having important effects on motivation for behavioural change in the various stages in the epidemic, depending on the social discourse and images associated with it. Information-related and cognitive factors have been found, for instance, to play a decisive role in the initial perception phase and to be less important at subsequent stages. In the same vein, Catania, Kegeles and Coates (1990) have proposed an AIDS risk reduction model (ARRM) that defines the pathway to individual behavioural change as consisting of three stages, *viz.*, recognizing and labelling one's sexual behaviours as high risk for contracting HIV, committing oneself to the idea that it is necessary to reduce this risk exposure, and actively searching for and implementing strategies to reach this goal. According to this approach, the individual and collective components liable to be involved in this process of behaviour change are expected to vary in each of these three stages. The most interesting feature here is not so much the model itself, but the fact that the authors state explicitly that no attempt will be made to search for causal determinants, since the 'proposed model stands as an heuristic device intended to facilitate the conceptual organization of research on individual behaviour change, and intervention development and evaluation' (Catania, Kegeles and Coates, 1990).

We share to a great extent these American colleagues' conviction that social science work on explanatory theories of HIV-related risk behaviours must free itself from the mechanistic conception of causality that has prevailed to date. From the technical point of view, we are convinced that a more diversified use of statistical multidimensional methods for analysing empirical data (such as giving more space to factor analysis) could be a helpful step in that direction.

Large-scale surveys on sexual behaviour, such as the ACSF study carried out in France and its English and American equivalents, have provided an exceptionally vast amount of data that has served to identify the factors involved in exposure to the risk of sexual HIV transmission more accurately and in greater detail than was previously possible. From now on it seems to be of the utmost importance that no further illusory deterministic searching should go on in making use of these data, but that the emphasis should be placed on investigating specific contexts and individual histories more closely. We feel it is also essential that thought be given in the future to ways of achieving greater complementarity between quantitative and qualitative approaches so that there will be less danger of veering from the one to the other for no particular reason apart from the random dictates of fashion.

In this chapter our standpoint has been basically that of insiders with some experience of this particular kind of research taking a critical look at the limitations of the behavioural models that have been applied to HIV prevention up to now. Other authors in their contributions to this volume have proposed to sum up the situation on the basis of more fundamental social science research on human sexuality. This should provide a good basis for assessing the weaknesses of behavioural models from the outside, which we are convinced is as badly needed as the approach we ourselves have adopted here.

Appendix 1: An Application of the Expected Utility Model to the Decision to Use Condoms

The idea of expected utility was first introduced by Bernouilli to solve the well-known paradox about the Saint Petersburg game. By hypothesizing that the gamblers were attempting to maximize the expected utility of their gains, Bernouilli not only solved the paradox, but also laid the foundations for modern decision theory. At a much later date von Neuman and Morgenstern (1947) used this concept of expected utility as the basis of an axiomatic theory about the rational choices made by an individual who has to decide between several alternative actions, the results of which cannot be predicted with certainty. Here expected utility means the subjective quality or satisfaction which an individual hopes to maximize in terms of mathematical expectation, i.e., the product of the probability that an outcome will occur multiplied by the magnitude or value attached to this outcome by the individual.

In the diagram in Figure 6.1 this model is applied to the decision as to whether or not a condom should be used during one sexual encounter. To simplify the decision tree we have assumed that only one of the two partners is able to decide for both of them and that the other possible advantages of using a condom for protection from HIV (such as protection from other STDs and contraception) are not taken into account (because the female partner is taking oral contraception, for example). It is also assumed (although this of course is overly optimistic) that the condom affords 100 per cent protection from infection; finally, it is assumed that the person taking the decision is seronegative.

The model simply shows that condom use is a rational choice if and only if its expected utility for the individual decision-maker exceeds that of the alternative option (no condoms). As can be seen from Figure 6.1, this expected utility calculation will depend first on how the individual assesses the two probabilities, that is, the probability (p) that his partner may carry the HIV virus and the probability (q) that intercourse may lead to transmission of the disease if the partner does in fact carry the virus.

However, the expected utility will depend not only on this probabilistic risk assessment, but also on other values (or utilities) the individual associates with the possible outcomes of his decision. The individual decision-maker actually has to judge between the greatest benefit likely to be derived from sexual intercourse without worrying about the disadvantages of using a condom or about the consequences of HIV infection if no condom is used. It seems logical, moreover, to assume that the individual will tend to classify the values he associates with the various possible outcomes by ranking them from *best* (having intercourse with no condom without being infected) to *worst* (becoming HIV-infected), with the relative desirability of having intercourse with a condom and no HIV infection being given an intermediate rating.

References

AGRAFIOTIS, D. (Ed.) (1989) 'Knowledge, attitudes, beliefs and practices, in relation to HIV infection and AIDS, The Case of the City of Athens', Athens: Department of Sociology, Athens School of Public Health, WHO.

AGRAFIOTIS, D. (Ed.) (1991) 'Technical and statistical support in the comparative and in depth analysis of data collected through KABP studies funded by GPA/WHO: The Cases of Togo and Mauritins', Department of Sociology, Research Monographs, 7, Athens School of Public Health.

ALLAIS, M. (1953) 'Le comportement de l'homme rationnel devant le risque: Critique des postulats et axiomes de l'école américaine', *Econometrica*, **21**, pp. 503–46.

ARCHER, V.E. (1988) 'Psychological defenses and control of AIDS', *American Journal of Public Health*, **79**, pp. 876–8.

ARRAS, J.D. (1990) 'AIDS and reproductive decisions: Having children in fear and trembling', *Milbank Quarterly*, **68**, pp. 353–82.

AUGÉ, M. and HERZLICH, C. (1984) 'Le Sens du Mal', *Anthropologie, Histoire, Sociologie de la Maladie*, Paris: Editions des Archives Contemporaine.

BANDURA, A. (1977) 'Self-efficacy: Toward a unifying theory of behavioral change', *Psychological Review*, **84**, pp. 191–215.

BECKER, M.H. (1974) 'The health belief model and personal health behavior', *Health Education Monographs*, **2**, pp. 220–43.

BECKER, M.I.L. and JOSEPH, J.G. (1988) 'AIDS and behavioral change to reduce risk: A review', *American Journal of Public Health*, **78**, pp. 394–410.

BLENDON, R.J., DONELAN, K. and KNOX, R.A. (1992) 'Public opinion and AIDS: Lessons from the second decade', *Journal of American Medical Association*, **267**, pp. 981–6.

BOUDON, R. (1979) *La Logique du Social: Introduction à l'Analyse Sociologique*, Paris: Hachette.

CATANIA, J.A., KEGELES, S.M. and COATES, T.J. (1990) 'Towards an understanding of risk behavior: An AIDS risk reduction model (ARRM)', *Health Education Quaterly*, **17**, pp. 53–72.

COATES, T.J. (1990) 'Strategies for modifying sexual behavior for primary and secondary prevention of HIV disease', *Journal of Consulting and Clinical Psychology*, **58**, pp. 57–69.

COATES, T.J. and GREENBLATT, R.M. (1989) 'Behavioral change using community level interventions', in HOLMES, K. (Ed.) *Sexually Transmitted Diseases*, New York: McGraw-Hill.

COATES, T.J., STALL, R.D., Catania, J.A. and KEGELES, S. (1988) 'Behavioral factors in HIV infection', *AIDS*, **2** (1), pp. 239–46.

COHEN, D.R. and MOONEY, G.H. (1984) 'Prevention goods and hazard goods: A taxonomy', *Scottish Journal of Political Economy*, **31**, pp. 92–9.

COHEN, M. (1991) 'Designing AIDS prevention programs based on three frameworks explaining sexual behaviour change in gay populations', in JOB-SPIRA, N., SPENCER, B., MOATTI, J.P. and BOUVET, E. (Eds) *Santé Publique et Maladie à Transmission Sexuelle*, Paris: John Libbey Eurotext.

DAVIES, P.M., WEATHERBURN, P. and HICKSON, F.C.I. (1993) 'Science, gay men and AIDS: New directions for research', presentation at the 9th International Conference on AIDS, Berlin, June (WS-D07-6).

DAVISON, C., DAVEY, C., DAVIES, P. and FRANKEL, S. (1991) 'Lay epidemiology and the prevention paradox: The implications of coronary candidary for health education', *Sociology of Health and Illness*, **13**, pp. 1–19.

DE VROOME, E.M.M., PAALMAN, M.E.M. SANFORT, TH.G.M. SLEUTJES, M., DEVRIES, K.J.M. and TIELMAN, R. (1990) 'AIDS in the Netherlands: The effects of several years of campaigning', *International Journal of Sexually Transmitted Diseases and AIDS*, **1**, pp. 268–75.

DOWNIE, R.S., FIFE, C. and TANNAHILL, A. (1991) *Health Promotion: Models and Values*, Oxford: Oxford University Press.

DUBOIS-ARBER, F., LEHMANN, P.H., HAUSSER, D., ZIMMERMAN, E. and GUTZWILLER, F. (1989) 'Evaluation des campagnes de prévention du SIDA en Suisse: Deuxième rapport de synthèse', Cahiers de recherche, Document IUMSP 39, Lausanne.

EKSTRAND, M. and COATES, T. (1990) 'Maintenance of safer sexual behaviors and predictors of risky sex: The San Francisco's Men's Health Study', *American Journal Public Health*, **80**, pp. 973–7.

EKSTRAND M., STALL, R., MALATT, A., POLLACK, G.L., McKUSICK, L. and COATES, T. (1992) 'Frequent and infrequent relapsers need different AIDS prevention programs', presentation at The 8th International Conference on AIDS, Amsterdam, July.

ELSTER, J. (1979) *Ulysses and the Sirens*, Cambridge: Cambridge University Press.

FISCHHOFF, B., LICHTENSTEIN, S., SLOVIC, P., DERBY, S.L. and KEENEY, R.L. (1981) *Acceptable Risk*, New York: Cambridge University Press.

HAUSSER, D., LEHMANN, P., SOMANI, B. and GUTZWILLER, F. (1987) 'Evaluation des campagnes nationales de prévention contre le SIDA: modèle d'analyse', *Soz Praeventivmed*, **32**, pp. 207–9.

HAUSSER, D., LEHMANN, P., ZIMMERMAN, E. and GUTZWILLER, F. (1988) 'Effectiveness of the AIDS prevention campaigns in Switzerland', in *The Global Impact of AIDS*, New York: Alain R. Liss.

HAUSSER, D., ZIMMERMAN, E. and DUBOIS-ARBER, F. (1991) 'Evaluation of the AIDS prevention strategy in Switzerland: Third assessment report (1989–1990)', Lausanne: Institut Universitaire de médecine sociale et préventive. (Cahiers de recherches, Document IUMSP 52b.)

HELLINGER, F.J. (1989) 'Expected utility theory and risk choices with health outcomes', *Medical Care*, **27**, pp. 273–9.

HORNUNG, R., HELMINGER, A. and HATTICH, A. (1992) *AIDS in Bewusstsein der Bevölk-erung*, Zürich: ISPM.

HOMAR, P.M. and KAHLE, L.R. (1988) 'A structural equation test of the value-attitude-behavior hierarchy', *Journal of Personality and Social Psychology*, **54**, pp. 638–46.

JANZ, N.K. and BECKER, M.H. (1984) 'The health belief model: A decade later', *Health Education Quarterly*, **11**, pp. 1–47.

JOB, R.F.S. (1988) 'Effective and ineffective use of fear in health promotion campaigns', *American Journal of Public Health*, **78**, pp. 163–7.

JODELET, D. (1989) (Ed.) *Les Représentations Sociales*, Paris: Presses universitaires françaises.

KELLY, J., LAWRENCE, J., SMITH, S., HOOD, H.V. and COOK, D.J. (1987) 'Stigmatization of AIDS patients by physicians', *American Journal of Public Health*, **77**, pp. 789–91.

KRASINSKI, K., BORKOWSKY, W., BEBENROTH, D. and MOORE, T. (1988) 'Failure of voluntary testing for HIV to identify infected parturient women in a high risk population', *New England Journal of Medicine*, **318**, pp. 185.

LEHMANN, P., HAUSSER, D., SOMAINI, B. and GUTZWILLER, F. (1987) 'Campaign against AIDS in Switzerland: Evaluation of a nationwide educational programme', *British Medical Journal*, **295**, pp. 1118–20.

LEVENTHAL, L.H. (1973) 'Changing attitudes and habits to reduce risk factors in chronic disease', *American Journal of Cardiology*, **31**, pp. 571–80.

LEVITON, J.C. (1989) 'Theorical foundations of AIDS-prevention programs', in VALDISERRI, R.O. (Ed.) *Preventing AIDS: The Design of Effective Programs*, New Brunswick and London: Rutgers University Press.

LINDENBERG, S. (1985) 'An assessment of the new political economy: Its potential for the social sciences and sociology in particular', *Sociological Theory*, **3**, pp. 99–114.

LOOMES, G. and SUGDEN, R. (1982) 'Regret theory: An alternative theory of rational choice under uncertainty', *Economic Journal*, **92**, pp. 805–24.

MANN, J. and KAY, K. (1988) 'Sida discrimination et santé publique', presentation at The IVth International Conference on AIDS, Stockholm, June.

MASUR, J.B. and DUBOIS-ARBER, F. (1990) 'Evaluation de la stratégie de prévention du Sida en Suisse: Homosexuels', Cahiers de recherche, Document IUMSP 52.8, Lausanne.

MOATTI, J.P. (1991) 'Les enquêtes sur les connaissances, attitudes, croyances et pratiques face au Sida: Usage et usure d'un outil', *Journal du Sida*, **31** (32), pp. 21–6.

MOATTI, J.P. and SERRAND, C. (1989) 'Les sciences sociales face au Sida: Entre silence et trop parler?', *Cahiers de Sociologie et de Démographie Médicales*, **3**, pp. 231–62.

MOATTI, J.P., DAB, W., LOUNDOU, H., QUENEL, P., BELTZER, W., ANÈS, A. and POLLACK, M. (1992) 'Impact on the general public of media campaigns against AIDS: A French evaluation', *Health Policy*, **21**, pp. 233–47.

MOATTI, J.P., DAB, W., POLLAK, M. and GROUPE KABP FRANCE (1992) 'Les Français et le Sida', *La Recherche*, **23**, pp. 1202–11.

MOATTI, J.P., LE GALES, C., SEROR, V., PAPIERNIK, E. and HENRION, R. (1990) 'Social acceptability of HIV screening among pregnant women', *AIDS Care*, **2**, pp. 213–22.

PESCOSOLIDO, B.A. (1992) 'Beyond rational choice: The social dynamics of how people seek help', *American Journal of Sociology*, **4**, pp. 1096–138.

POLLAK, M. (Ed.) (1988) *Les Homosexuels et le Sida, Sociologie d'une Epidémie*, Paris: A. Métaillié.

ROSENBERG, M.L., TOUSMA, D.D., KOLBE, L.J., KRUGER, F., CYNAMON, M.L. and BOWEN, S.G. (1992) 'The role of behavioral sciences and health education in HIV prevention (Experience at the US Center for Disease Control)', in SEPULVEDA, J., FINEBERG, H. and MANN, J. (Eds) *AIDS Prevention Through Education: A World View*, New York: Oxford University Press.

SLOVIC, P., FISCHHOFF, B. and LICTENSTEIN, S. (1980) 'Facts and fears: Understanding perceived risk', in SCHWEIG, C. and ALBERS, W.A. (Eds) *Societal Risk Assessment*, New-York: Plenum Press.

SOLAMAR, M.Z. and DEJONG, W. (1986) 'Recent STD's prevention efforts and their implications for AIDS health education', *Health Education Quaterly*, **13**, pp. 301–16.

STIFFMAN, A.R. (1991) 'Change in AIDS behaviors from adolescence to adulthood', presentation at The 7th International Conference on AIDS, June, Florence (WD1).

STOLLER, E.J. and RUTHERFORD, G.W. (1989) 'Evaluation of AIDS prevention and control program', *AIDS*, **3**, supplement 1, pp. 289–96.

TURNER, M. (1982) 'Toward a cognitive redefinition of the social group', in TAJFEL, H. (Ed.) *Social Identity and Intergroup Relation*, Cambridge: Cambridge Uiversity Press.

TVERSKY, A. and KAHNEMAN, D. (1974) 'Judgment under uncertinty: Heuristics and biases', *Science*, **185**, pp. 1124–31.

TYMSTRA, T. (1989) 'The imperative character of medical technology and the meaning of anticipated decision regret', *International Journal of Technology Assessment in Health Care*, **5**, pp. 601–18.

VON NEUMANN, J. and MORGENSTERN, O. (1947) *Theories of Games and Economic Behavior*, Princeton: Princeton University Press.

Chapter 7

From Rational Individual to Actor Ensnared in a Web of Affective and Sexual Relationships

Benoît Bastard and Laura Cardia-Vonèche

Introduction

How one should analyse the ways individuals cope with the risk of AIDS in their relationships is one of the keys for prevention and a major challenge for the social sciences. So far, many of the efforts made by investigators have led to dead ends. It is still difficult to be able to account for and predict individuals' behaviour systematically when it comes to talking about AIDS or managing the risk of HIV infection. Even informed persons who profess preventive attitudes do not comply in practice with the very principles to which they subscribe when it comes to protection, or they vary their behaviour from one relationship to the next.

The difficulties that are encountered may prompt one to give up the search for rational explanations. Behaviour in the realm of emotions and sex apparently cannot be broken down to cause-and-effect relationships. The fact that individuals are guided by their emotions, desires, even fantasies, makes all systematic analysis of their behaviour in the emotion-charged realm of sexuality difficult and prediction of their behaviour problematic. Still, many investigations strive to uncover what drives individuals in this area. To do this, they expand the analysis of the links between attitudes and behaviour by including ever more sophisticated parameters, or try to show that the individual harbours a fleet of rationalities that may conflict with each other, thereby explaining the variability of behaviour or deviations from expected behaviour.

The question nevertheless remains unanswered: Can one reach a satisfactory explanation while remaining within the confines of a theory that posits that decisions about how to cope with health risks are made by rational

individuals? Must not we change our perspective and switch from an analysis of the rational subject to analysis of the rationality of interactions? These questions are discussed in this chapter.[1]

The heart of the matter is the validity of individual-oriented analysis. How do we describe the individual? How do we perceive the motivations behind their actions? What are the possibilities of influencing them? In our opinion, clear answers to these questions are necessary for both research and prevention. That is why we shall tackle the issue in two stages, first, by recalling the individual-oriented research that has been conducted to date and the criticism levelled at this type of explanation of behaviour, then developing an alternative that consists in resituating the subject in his or her web of interactions and relationships and describing the logic of his or her interactions.

Criticism of Individual-based Models

Earlier in this section Moatti, *et al.*, and Ingham and van Zessen each describe individual-oriented models that hypothesize that strong cause-and-effect relationships link individual knowledge of, attitudes toward, and behaviour with respect to the risk of AIDS. These variables characterize individuals' knowledge and attitudes – 'knowing, feeling or evaluating' (Ahlemeyer and Ludwig) – and cover a wide range of factors including individuals' knowledge of the disease and its routes of transmission; their assessments of the risk; their intentions with regard to prevention; their abilities, learning aptitudes, and their ability to put the intentions they express into effect. The variables that characterize risk-related behaviour (acting) basically boil down to the adoption of or failure to adopt preventive behaviour or placing oneself in what are defined as at-risk situations based on current medical knowledge.

The supporters of models such as the Health Belief Model – a prime example of an individual-based model – take it for granted that advances in knowledge and the acquisition of the right attitudes and new abilities are the ways to acquire risk-avoiding preventive behaviour. Such assumptions are not totally unfounded, at least in appearance. They account for certain quantitative survey data fairly well and there seem to be certain links between the socio-demographic variables that are associated with a low level of health education and the risk of HIV infection. Studies also underline that the more the condom is seen as ineffectual, the less it is used. However, according to the authors who have reported such findings (Moatti, *et al.*), they result from flaws in the research design or interpretation of the results. Either the separation between dependent and independent variables is not truly made and the analysis remains largely tautological, or the observers are mistaken about the direction of the causal link. The knowledge displayed by individuals may not cause health-related behaviour but, on the contrary, individuals may use the knowledge at their disposal to justify their behaviour after the fact. In such a case, a link between attitudes and behaviour does exist, but its direction is misconstrued. Clearly, the HBM overestimates people's rationality, at least if rationality is defined as the fact that these individuals adopt behaviour in line with their principles.

The criticism of individual-oriented models concerns quantitative and qualitative analysis. With regard to quantitative research, contrary to the limited examples given above, it is not certain that these models are validated by survey data, especially those that try to measure the effects of prevention campaigns. As suggested by Moatti, *et al.*, some analyses reveal rather illogical links between beliefs, attitudes and behaviour, and often the cause and effect remain illusory. As for qualitative analyses, the data presented by authors in this book completely invalidate hypotheses of a simple cause-and-effect relationship flowing from knowledge and attitudes to behaviour. The conceptual weakness of the individual-oriented model is demonstrated by the numerous examples cited where an individual has all the predispositions for engaging in safer behaviour but then continue risky behaviour. Ludwig and Ahlemeyer give the example of a woman who had all the trumps needed to adopt preventive behaviour but failed to play them. This prompted them to quip, 'AIDS has obviously changed a lot in heads but little in bed'. The discussion of the relapse issue suggests that people who have adopted safer behaviour that is apparently founded on preventive logic do not maintain such behaviour in the long term (Moatti, *et al.*). Upon reflection, Moatti notes that relapsing is part of a chain of different behaviours, each of which obeys a different logic. Finally, Ingham and van Zessen underline their failure to detect in the people they studied a learning process following their awareness of the errors they admitted having committed in the light of AIDS-prevention information.

The disparity between these results and our expectations of HBM-type models may be the result of flaws in design. One flaw is the assumption of *linearity*, where cognitive elements are often considered prerequisites for action, although they may just as well serve to legitimate actions. Another is that models do not allow for the complexity of decision-making. In some studies a single variable is associated with a single behaviour. Such an association is a gross simplification, especially when, as the critics claim, the choice of the variable is subject to field-related bias. Even when a larger number of pertinent variables is chosen, their arrangement in dichotomous categories (for example, the subject's intention or lack of intention to protect him or herself), fails to allow for the complexity or variability of individuals' behaviour and the diversity of their reactions in the various contexts in which they find themselves. Thus, such studies do not allow for the chain of elements involved in decision-making. Perhaps most importantly, many studies do not specify that the sexual decision involves the subject, his or her partner, and possibly other significant people, even anticipating what might occur during an interaction. Instead, they act as if risk assessment were specific to the individual. For example, Ingham and van Zessen hypothesize that when individuals imagine that their partners oppose condom use, their own intentions to use a condom will be greatly weakened. The intention to use a condom was fairly widespread in the sample these authors studied. If we took only the intention and not the possibility of such opposition into account we would overestimate the individuals' condom use greatly.

Based on the criticism levelled at HBM-type models, some authors have developed more refined analytical models. One example of such a model is the micro-economic utility model proposed by Moatti, *et al.*, who suggest that such an approach accounts better for the uncertainties that characterize the subject's calculations and that risk-taking is rational for the individual at certain times. This refined model is referred to the concept of limited rationality because the subject's information and means of calculation are imperfect. From a prevention perspective, this model suggests that improving individuals' information and ability to look ahead will improve the likelihood of their adopting safer sexual practices. This same model also suggests that the irrationality expressed by unsafe behaviour by people who have the proper knowledge about prevention is only apparent. These people may be driven by other motivations that are rational in areas outside the health sphere. What is more, there is tension between different rationalities. In such a perspective, an actor is caught between two lines of fire and forced to arbitrate between antagonistic logics. For example, the value given to continuing a relationship may be deemed sufficient for an individual who is highly motivated by preventive concerns to renounce practising prevention if he or she fears the chosen partner's reluctance. As noted in Bastard, *et al.* in chapter 3, a relative scarcity of potential partners and the level of expectations about a given relationship are relevant factors in such an approach. The choices that are made show that the person either sticks to his or her prevention principles or puts relations first. Because the revised models keep individuals at the decision-making centre, the issue is then whether one is better able to understand the individual's behaviour. Shouldn't we go beyond the actor's point of view and consider the matter of the interaction itself? If so, how is rationality involved?

Rationality and Irrationality of Behaviour

The conception of the individual that emerges from this book is complex because it blends rational elements with those that do not seem to be rational when it is assumed that individuals are at the centre of their universe. In practice, individuals are caught in various contexts; they are driven by differentiated and changing incentives, and their opportunities are as important to the individual as principles. For example, in an interaction described by

Ingham and van Zessen, the fact that a couple has condoms in the car's glove compartment (and not in the commode drawer, ten feet away) appears to be a decisive factor in determining whether to adopt this means of protection. Similarly, we deal with individuals who make adjustments, go through alternating phases of calculation, react to unforeseen situations, and make split-second decisions in the heat of the moment. Ludwig stresses the point that individuals are not scientists. Alongside their limited mathematical abilities they having enormous abilities to assimilate new data and adapt to situations. However, she emphasizes the importance of emotions and desire in these reactions and adjustments.

How can this sometimes rational, sometimes irrational (to the extent that it corresponds more to opportunities than to principles) functioning of the individual be theoretically described? Moatti, *et al.*, suggest one way at the end of their text. These authors offer the image of multifaceted individuals whose facets are activated by the situations in which they operate. This idea is tempting, for it accounts for the essential aspects of variability of behaviour and the lack of consistency observed in certain individuals. It might be more operational if some individuals are allowed to be multifaceted whereas others are one-dimensional. It also is complementary to the distinction between primary and secondary space that Peto, *et al.* (1992) apply to the issue of AIDS risk-related behaviour. In highlighting the fact that the applicable norms and risk management strategies differ according to the space considered and the types of relations that develop therein, these authors also account for differences in behaviour without assuming some inconsistent behaviours.

Another tempting framework is found in Ahlemeyer and Ludwig's text. These authors stress the need to ask *when* an individual is located in a given perspective rather than knowing *who* the individual truly is. In doing this they discourage the depiction of individuals with stable inclinations who have the same behaviour regardless of the context or partner.

Scripts are another avenue mentioned in passing in many of the chapters in this book. Individuals are guided by very powerful scripts that are specific to their cultures or groups. The use of this notion doubtless requires that the definition of scripts be refined and the way scripts link with the other perspectives presented by our contributors be specified (see Chapter 8 for example). Some relevant questions for describing the variability of behaviour include: Are the scripts in question so compelling that they allow individuals who belong to a given group to keep their distance from the reigning norm or, on the contrary, does the notion of a script include the idea that individuals appropriate the roles that are conferred on them and act them out?

Even with these revisions, however, Moatti underscores that this model is fundamentally the same as the HBM, and the emphasis on tensions between normative universes with sometimes converging, sometimes diverging, logics, fails to satisfy us. While reactions to conflicts of norms or interests do make it possible to reconstruct the rationality of certain behaviours, a cost/benefit model, even if it allows for several reference universes, still does not surmount the problems plaguing individual-oriented models. In these models, we are still grappling with the implicit idea that man is guided mainly by reason and searches for well-being in health matters by weighing such well-being against well-being in other areas (Ahlemeyer and Ludwig). This perspective does not allow sufficiently for the context where decisions do not rest solely with an individual but are the products of interactions to or with relationships. The Health Belief Model, like the other models mentioned above, may be useful for predicting behaviour in certain areas, but does not appear to be valid for analysing sexuality. In practice, sexuality is not a personal health problem. 'Defining sexual activity as an individual health issue imposes certain sets of constructs on the field, with the result that some crucial and essential elements of interactional processes are made invisible' (Ingham and van Zessen).

The Logic of the Interaction

Given the ways partners communicate about HIV infection and the ways they manage the AIDS risk in their sexual relations, we feel it is counterproductive to study the actors' behaviour independently of the stage on which the scene is being played. The logic of interaction, with its own characteristics and context, must be considered first and foremost. Ingham and van Zessen, for example, state, 'The actual outcomes depend to a large extent on interactional dynamics rather than on pre-existing attitudes.' They also stress that the partners themselves, even those with knowledge, abilities and experience, do not know how things will turn out. As they put it, 'People simply do not know what will happen in many situations.' The task becomes one of operationalizing this new perspective and many ways of doing it are proposed in the first section of this book.

Our own work suggests that protective behaviours are elements used in the partners' interaction. The building of such a relationship involves all sorts of signals that are exchanged by the partners. The partners must agree on the nature of the relationship and the type of investment it represents. Here verbal exchanges, unveiling intimacy, and other signs marking either attachment or boundaries set the scope of the exchange. Talking about AIDS, references to means of protection, and the actual use of condoms or tests function, in our view, as so many building blocks in the relationship-building process.

We see that a string of behaviours that are considered irrational from an individual-oriented perspective becomes consistent and understandable if considered an outcome of a relationship. This enables us to speak about the 'rationality of the relationship'. Ahlemeyer and Ludwig explore the systematic analysis where each intimate system has its own logic of action and generates its own norms and functions. Ferrand and Snijders have the same aim of revealing and conceptualizing the social network and the various types of logic that govern the relationship.

What Are the Implications for Prevention?

We started with the idea of a rational actor able to understand and put health principles into practice. Analysis of this first perspective led us to consider the idea of a complex, changing actor with regard to whom we can no longer talk about a single rationality, but various types of logics and incentives. A more fundamental break with these theories finally led us to consider the dynamics specific to affective and sexual relations.

According to this last approach, the behaviour that is adopted depends on the meaning that the interacting partners give to their relationship. This explains the transformations the same individual makes in the course of a given relationship or when moving from one relationship to the next. The meaning that is given to the relationship gradually crystallizes or changes with circumstances. This dynamic results in behaviours that do not appear to be connected and that may be entirely opposed to individuals' reported dispositions and attitudes. In developing this perspective we challenge some of the current foundations of prevention practices and, more broadly, the principles that govern education and teaching in our society. As we realize that other behavioural determinants beyond the individual's control and stemming from the logic of the situation are involved, the importance of the individual's responsibility and the individual's control over his or her environment and autonomy become less central. It thus remains for us to discuss the possible implications of such a switch in perspectives for prevention.

Prevention measures that exclusively spread information in order to change sexual behaviour are based on models that posit close links between knowledge and behaviour. This relationship is challenged in this text. By being limited to the rational sphere, it does not guarantee success, despite the fact that this is the only approach affording relatively easy access to the individual. This does not mean that disseminating information is useless, but merely that one must guard against establishing a direct connection with behaviour changes and not confine oneself to such campaigns. Alternative actions emerge as soon as one adopts a different perspective in which emphasis is placed on the interaction's logics rather than on the actor's rationality. The approach then becomes one of focusing prevention not on the individual, but on the system of interaction between partners and their networks. Here, however, the analytical approaches and types of intervention have still to be devised. Can one affect the social norms that govern the ways people enter into relationships so as to incorporate good practices as an indispensable way to start a relationship? Is it not a matter of acting upon the scripts mentioned above, focusing this time not on the actor, but on a scene involving several characters, that is, an interacting group? This is undoubtedly a difficult task, much more difficult than that of prevention aimed at a supposedly rational individual, but an indispensable one if we truly want to take up the issue of AIDS risk management.

Note

1 The summary presented in this chapter relies heavily on Ingham and van Zessen and Moatti *et al.*. We also considered some of the contributions made by Guizzardi and Stellla and Deven and Meredith.

Section III

Interaction and its Socio-cultural Context

Introduction

The third part of this book consists of three chapters. The first, by Deven and Meredith, provides a critical overview of Ira Reiss's comparative anthropology and shows its relevance to understanding sexual behaviour. Reiss's approach is used as a departure point for their own explanation of why individuals and partners adopt behaviours that place them at risk for HIV infection. Elements of other theoretical approaches, like the sexual scripts from Gagnon, complement Reiss's theory for a better articulation of the socio-cultural context and the actual interactions between the sexual partners.

The second chapter, by Guizzardi, Stella and Remy starts by criticizing the rationality which underlies preventive messages and is responsible for their relative ineffectiveness. They contrast this perspective with the idea of the construction of reality according to which legitimate messages result from a broad transaction–negotiation process in which various types of actors participate. With regard to microsocial phenomena, Guizzardi, Stella and Remy emphasize the importance of interactions within networks of significant others and peers in the production of effective norms and representations. They suggest that the media has a broad influence on defining these interactions. They also find that scientists who do research on HIV/AIDS or suggest prevention strategies are themselves significant actors in forming the public's images of AIDS and prevention.

One objective of this section is to advance the structuring and operationalizing of an interaction-oriented perspective started in the two previous introductory sections. Van Campenhoudt, in the last chapter of this section, first proposes a short overview of the theoretical field defined by the different perspectives presented in this book. He discusses the place and function of different sociological theories in elucidating sexual behaviour. From some examples of theoretical issues developed in this book, he shows how advancement and integration of theoretical is possible. Finally, he summarizes some methodological suggestions and issues in connexion with these theoretical perspectives.

Macro- and Microsocial Processes

The two first chapters suggest the influence that macrosocial conditions have over sexual behaviour. Sexuality has considerable importance in all societies, for it ensures the society's reproduction and binds the society's members to each other. Cultural norms regarding kinship, gender-based distribution of power and sexual ideology have specific functions to regulate sexual attitudes, beliefs and behaviours. Deven and Meredith's chapter expands upon the influence of macrosocial phenomena. For example, in Reiss's view, one function of marital jealousy is to discourage extramarital sex.

Regardless of the weight of these macrosocial conditions, the authors in this section warn against explaining sexual behaviour directly and mechanically by culture and culture's social functions. Macrosocial elements such as kinship patterns, power, social representations, etc., merely demarcate the probabilities of a behaviour in a given field where several scenarios can happen. The first reason for guarding against such mechanistic explanations is that the diversity and complexity of actual cultures and subcultures do not suggest the adoption of a uniform set of sexual behaviours or reactions to the risk of HIV infection. The symbols, values and norms that structure images of HIV/AIDS and sexuality are the results of complex processes of negotiations and transactions between various groups of actors with varying levels of influence. Many groups (doctors, scientists, prevention officers, moral, secular and religious authorities, the media, activist organizations, schools, families, etc.) act as gatekeepers. This negotiation–transaction process occurs continually in daily life. Consequently, its results are always unstable, temporary and often contradictory.

This is why individuals must arbitrate between these discourses and rearrange them to make their interpretations of messages coherent. According to Guizzardi, Stella, and Remy, who draw upon research conducted in Italy, individuals try to validate a certain image of themselves and, to this end, use the social resources that are within their reach. That means that in a sexual relationship partners interpret the socio-cultural context and are active participants in composing the boundaries of their own behaviour. The result is often that the same HIV/AIDS prevention message takes on different meanings and leads to different perceptions of the same risk. This relative autonomy is a second reason why the sexual behaviour of partners cannot be explained directly and mechanically by cultural and macrosocial factors. Deven and Meredith, for their part, use Gagnon's theory of scripts as a springboard for discussing this question.

Guizzardi, Stella and Remy consider social networks to be the social arenas in which macro- and microsocial processes complement each other. Norms generally accepted by society, medical and religious authorities' recommendations and prevention messages are used as references for the representations and experiences that prevail in interpersonal groups. The importance of relationship networks in small groups is fundamental in processes where individuals establish their own sexual boundaries. When such norms and recommendations are adopted, it is usually after being re-interpreted and reworked in a specific manner. Inversely, the norms and representations that are in force in these groups are challenged by the collective messages of influential others and the media and may be reworked through internal interactions in the groups. The individual's convictions and resolutions are forged through these interactions with their reference groups. This is where the most decisive social control occurs and, according to Ferrand and Snijders, most of the actual (rather than ideal) norms and sexual behaviour patterns take shape. This is where individuals use their margin of autonomy *vis-à-vis* social and cultural pressure, in their interactions and deliberations with others.

In explaining sexual behaviour we have noted the importance of societal norms and how they are interpreted and negotiated between their gatekeepers. They are, in turn, transferred to their groups, who reinterpret them to fit their own needs and preconceived views of the world. This two-step flow is indispensable, and the effective representations of norms and behaviour patterns bring us much closer to actual behaviour than individual-oriented perspectives. Still, it does not permit a direct explanation of sexual behaviour. They form a symbolic, normative and cognitive framework for the sexual relationship and an array of resources for the partners, but cannot account for the interactions that will take place at the heart of an intimate relationship. This means that specific conceptual frameworks must account for what happens in the relationship itself. This can be done only by establishing connections between formal explanations such as the social system theory and various material explanations for the specific interactions between partners.

As Van Campenhoudt shows in Chapter 10, one of the major conclusions of this book is that the various levels of social reality must not be studied as hierarchical. Throughout this book the view of vertical, one-way causality between macrosocial processes, microsocial processes and individual behaviours is challenged. The authors clearly see the social system as a whole, the various levels and structures of which must be distinguished, have relative autonomy and influence each other reciprocally and circularly.

Scientists, Doctors and Researchers as Actors (in Contrast to Invisible Observers)

Scientists and researchers are actors in the discourse on HIV/AIDS and their work reflects different perspectives and norms. Their approaches to problems are themselves social phenomena that can be studied. So, Guizzardi, Stella and Remy's criticism of the rational individual is not based on theoretical grounds alone, but also draws upon the sociology of knowledge. Different schools of science bring different constructs to their interpretation of HIV/ AIDS-related behaviour. For example, medical and health professionals will typically think – wrongly, according to our authors – that all individuals will actively make sacrifices to protect their health and improve their life expectancies if they are convinced that their lives are at stake. Similarly, economists typically hold that individuals tackle all problems of their existence as if they were optimization problems. Deven and Meredith make similar remarks. They note that in Reiss's theory the link between sexuality and the science of sexuality must be stated more clearly. Specifically, we must ask how science helps build its own subject of analysis or alters the phenomena that enter its field of analysis.

As in all fields, not everyone in the sciences has the same legitimacy or power. Some are more likely than others to have their views and perspectives accepted, to define their tasks themselves and to impose additional tasks on others. That is why Guizzardi, *et al.*, think that the social scientists should not let other categories of actors dictate what they should do, such as checking whether medical messages have been understood correctly by individuals. Rather, they should select their own tasks, such as trying to understand the process of producing and transforming legitimate representations of HIV/ AIDS.

Structure, Process and Meaning

In reviewing the debates about the holistic and functionalist nature of Reiss's approach, Deven and Meredith look for other theoretical avenues that would be better able to account for the actancial and dynamic dimensions of sexual behaviour when confronted by the risk of AIDS. To this end they discuss the merits of Gagnon's sexual scripts theory. They show that this approach makes it possible to account for social and cultural learning processes without holding individuals to be passive and uncritical.

Guizzardi, *et al.*, also refer very clearly to an actancial explanation that applies to both the macrosocial level and the microsocial level of interactions in networks of family and friends. It refers just as clearly to hermeneutic explanations that consist in revealing the *signified* from a set of *signifiers* by means of which they can be understood. This perspective is close to that of Bastard, *et al.*, according to whom the use or non-use of a condom (the signifier) can be interpreted to be a language that expresses what the relationship means to the partners (the signified). However, it appears even more forcefully here when our authors stress both the symbolic dimension of the representations of sexuality and risk and the meaning that the actors generate and give to their experiences. The complexity of images and meanings that they report contrasts with the simplicity of the image of the rational actor.

Finally, some of the arguments in this section stem from a dialectic approach. The main objective of the dialectic approach is to explain phenomena by focusing on internal contradictions in the phenomena under study. For example, it asks how individuals resolve the contradiction between pleasure and death in sexuality connected to HIV/AIDS or the contradiction between the positive image given to hedonism and the calls for sexual caution in the media. As a result, the dialectic explanation necessarily includes a dynamic process in the study of sexual behaviour. In other words, sexual behaviour can be understood by determining its place in the dialectic process that has to be reconstituted over time. The following three chapters complete our review of the various ways of explaining human and social reality; the systemic, functional and actancial explanations are here completed by the hermeneutic and dialectic explanations of sexual behaviour related to HIV/AIDS.

Chapter 8

The Relevance of a Macrosociological Perspective on Sexuality for an Understanding of the Risks of HIV Infection

Fred Deven and Philip Meredith

Introduction

This chapter considers the implications of reviews of the social anthropological and macrosociological perspective on human sexuality. Our analysis relates essentially to the approach offered by Ira L. Reiss as it has evolved from his 1986b study, *Journey into Sexuality.*[1] Reiss's work (and critical reactions to it) is of particular interest because his societal-level explanation of human sexuality combines comparative and interactionist sociology and cultural anthropology in describing how sexuality knits into the social fabric. These disciplines are seen as very much alike in their macro-level approach and within this context offer insights into sexual behaviours and attitudes related to the risk of HIV/AIDS. This approach must be able to provide a detailed account of the risk behaviour of European youth while not losing touch with the epidemiological reality of HIV transmission, which is transcontinental and is likely to be increasingly related to the contact between modern and traditional societies in transition.

Background

A range of perspectives exist that may be used to make sense of the origin and influence of human sexuality, and there is a danger in ignoring any single primary frame of reference. The most common frames of reference are societal institutions, physiological processes and individual experiences. Commonalities across different approaches or paradigms indicate that scholars view certain issues as central to understanding human sexuality (Geer and O'Donohue, 1987). In his review of sociological perspectives on human sexuality, Delamater (1987) has contended that sociologists have failed to attempt any truly comprehensive analysis. Thus, most of the research and theoretical models emerging from the sociological perspective are believed to have focused on specific types of sexual expression such as pre- and extra-marital sexuality, homosexuality and female prostitution, at the expense of the general phenomenon.

In reviewing human sexuality from the anthropological perspective, social scientists must make a distinction between descriptive and comparative cultural anthropology. Davenport (1987) adopts a strong culturally-relativist point of view in his notion of *cultures of sex* to specify the social or institutional contexts within which all behaviour related to sexuality occurs. He stresses that these cultures of sex are extremely variable in terms of ideologies and values. A culture of sex establishes two kinds of environment within which sexuality is transformed into behaviour: one is ideational and normative, the other is social and regulatory. Davis and Whitten (1987) suggest that more emphasis be placed on combining studies of heterosexual practices with studies of gender and symbolism in order to incorporate the erotic and pleasure dimensions of sex. Moreover, they consider that the typologies of sexually-restrictive and sexually-permissive societies are ethnocentric and obscure the socio-cultural complexity of sexual behaviour in a particular setting. By contrast, they see anthropological research on homosexual rather than heterosexual behaviour is seen as being grounded in its own social, domestic, religious and political contexts.

Recent reviews related to HIV/AIDS-relevant research and the anthropological perspective have proposed that greater emphasis be given to the descriptive-ethnographic data. Carrier and Bolton (1991), for example, make three types of recommendations in this respect: First, basic ethnographic study should be done on the hidden vectors of HIV transmission, particularly in sexual behaviour and IV drug use. Second, descriptive data should be collected on the effects of sexual orientation, especially on gay or bisexual youth. Third, research should be done on developmentally related areas of risk across the life span.

Against this background, Reiss's contribution builds on comparative anthropology to develop these theoretical proposals, choosing an ethnological approach to best elucidate the extent of cultural variation. *Journey into Sexuality* (1986b) aims to provide a scholarly, integrated, societal-level explanation of human sexuality. The author therefore chooses to emphasize those universal societal features that are linked to a wide range of sexual customs. His focus is upon societal linkages, leaving to others the task of developing connections to other areas, such as physiology, psychology or politics. He asserts that none of the existing schema, for example, orthodox Freudian psychology, Marxism, sociobiology, allow for adequate explanation of why people in various societies have such different sexual lifestyles.

Reiss's Concepts and Assumptions

It is acknowledged that, in the English language, the term *sex* is used with three distinct meanings, namely: as the genetic sex, as referring to a gender role, and as an act such as intercourse. For the sake of scientific precision, Reiss (1989) proposes to employ the term *human sexuality* to refer specifically, in sociological terms, to 'the erotic arousal and genital responses resulting from following the shared sexual scripts of that society'.

The following constitutes some of the explicit assumptions underpinning his theoretical explanation:

- The scientific approach is one way to understand social reality. Science is referred to as systematized knowledge based upon observation and experimentation that is directed toward explaining and predicting the phenomenon studied.
- All human behaviour is self-oriented. It is motivated by the pursuit of pleasure and the avoidance of pain. Reiss takes a modified version of hedonism in human behaviour by asserting that people's selves vary in the degree to which they incorporate the welfare of others as a source of pleasure and pain.
- Societal-level causes are major influences on our sexual life-styles. Hence, in the examination of life-styles of societies or groups, sociology is clearly central to any explanation.

The Social Importance of Sexuality

Reiss documents the social nature of human sexuality, asserting that it is given importance in all societies, regardless of the level of sexual permissiveness, because it is related mainly to physical pleasure and self-disclosure. All societies, in their customs, either by direct praise or radical attempts to control, pay tribute to the physical pleasure potential in sexual relationships. As sexuality alters our state of mind, it promotes self-disclosure. This refers to revealing an aspect of oneself that is not generally exposed. Disclosure may lead to the development of affection or closeness in feeling. According to Reiss, physical pleasure and disclosure in all societies are to be viewed as generic building blocks of sexual relationships. However, 'Neither of these characteristics is guaranteed to accompany every sexual act, nor will the presence of either always be maximal' (Reiss, 1986b).

In his cross-cultural examination of human sexuality, Reiss identifies three features of a society that stamp sexuality most deeply, namely, kinship, power, and ideology (though not the entirety of each of these areas is centrally linked to sexuality). In making sense of human sexuality he contends that marital sexual jealousy is the focal point in kinship relations, power is manifested most clearly in gender roles, and ideology expresses what is considered sexual normality for any group.

Kinship

Beginning with the institutionalized area of the kinship system, each society sets boundaries for important relationships, such as the marital relationship, in which people are expected to invest themselves deeply. The norms of all societies usually stress, to a lesser or greater extent, affection, duty, and pleasure as the three key reasons for marital sexual boundaries. Western societies stress the importance of love.

The systemic linkage to kinship is most easily illustrated in the area of marital jealousy. Considered from a sociological or group perspective, it is a boundary-maintaining mechanism for what the group feels are important relationships. Following this view, those sexual relationships which are considered important are predominantly ringed with the alarm system of jealousy, which tends to restrict those additional relationships that are thought to be disruptive of kinship and friendship ties.

The strength of jealousy varies greatly within different societies, as does the specific sexual relationships which arouse jealousy. One major explanation of cultural differences in marital sexual jealousy asserts that the greater the male's power, the stronger the husband's sexual jealousy. Societies in which wives hold more power will tend to be correspondingly more egalitarian.

Social Power

Compared with the above, the systemic linkage of sexuality to power is more obvious for Reiss. Because sexuality is an important aspect of social life and since the powerful by definition are those who are able to obtain the largest share of whatever they wish, it is then argued that the powerful will have freer access to sexuality than the powerless. In Western societies men have more power than women in virtually all major institutions (economics, politics, religion). The sexual customs of our society still demand more control over and condemnation of female than male sexuality. Following this reasoning, we propose that it is unlikely that one can have full sexual equality without equality in the domain of institutional power.

The power of each gender is the key influence on the sexual scripts of that gender. For example, Reiss's cross-cultural research indicates that two factors – the presence of a macho male role and a belief that females are inferior – are the best predictors of rape rates in diverse societies. It is interesting that Reiss finds that such societies have the highest rates of male homosexual behaviour. Two explanations are provided for this finding. First, the narrower the shared conception of any social role, the fewer the number of people who will be able to comply and will be interested in complying. Second, the feeling of being out of step with the cultural requirements of the male role may have an impact on one's sexual orientation. This second proposition is valid predominantly for males living in societies where homosexuality is viewed as opposed to heterosexuality.

Ideology

The third systemic linkage to our sexual life-styles is ideology, more specifically the notions of sexual normality and abnormality. The use of these terms is often an expression of group value positions that can be raised to the mythical level of scientific labels. Reiss asserts that our notions of sexual abnormality will largely support the views of these kin and power elements. The author prefers to distinguish (hetero)sexual ideologies in terms of the degree of gender equality, spelling out four basic perspectives that distinguish the egalitarian from the non-egalitarian sexual ideology. The first tenet concerns the endorsement of gender equality in the key institutional areas of a society; the second concerns body-centred sexuality; the third the degree of addiction to, and fear associated with, sexuality; and the fourth, the major goal(s) of sexuality.[2] Noticing the differential gender sequencing of social changes that occurred in the West during the last two decades, we conclude that the egalitarian sexual ideology will become dominant in the future.

In sum, it is asserted that all societies view sexuality as important because they recognize its potential for interpersonal bonding and are concerned with who bonds with whom. Western societies are particularly concerned about marriage and so erect strong jealousy norms around marriage to monitor any unwanted sexual bonding. Those in power will tend to acquire the rights of control over sexuality at the expense of those without power. This has significance for gender relationships, which usually are male-dominated, and will affect the nature of sexual interaction. The sexual customs that develop in accordance with the above constraints tend to be embodied in the beliefs about abnormality; individuals will feel compelled to adhere to those beliefs.

Major Propositions

In his 1986b work Reiss offered a propositional structure of his macrosociological theory of human sexuality. This is organized in order to make his theoretical structure act as a basis for his theory, research and predicting sexual behaviour. Twenty-five propositions, organized within four areas, comprise the basic logical and propositional structure. Each proposition is qualified with a *ceteris paribus* (assuming that all else is equal). Each of the four theoretical areas starts with broad general propositions drawn from specific empirical data that serve as the premises for some other propositions in that set.[3] The following propositions are formulated:

P1   Sexual bonding as the antecedent of kinship and gender roles. For example: Societies judge stable social relationships to be of great importance. Societies view physical pleasure and self-disclosure as the building blocks of stable social relationships. Physical pleasure and self-disclosure are the common outcomes of sexual behaviour. Therefore, sexual behaviour will be seen as important due to its ability to promote stable relationships.

P2   Sexuality and the power of each gender. For example: The authorized power of a group is basically utilized to obtain valued social goals. Therefore, since sexuality is a valued social goal, as a group gains power there will be increased sexual privileges in that group's sexual scripts, its erotica, and its ability to avoid sexual abuse.

P3   Ideology and sexuality. For example: Ideologies reflect and reinforce the social values operative in each of the major institutions. Therefore, to the extent that a gender's dominance is structured into the operant values of the basic institutions, ideologies will support the greater power of that gender and assign it greater rights in those institutional areas. General ideologies of a culture will be productive of specific sexual ideologies that reflect compatible ideological assumptions. Therefore, in a culture where one gender is dominant in the general ideology, that gender will be granted greater sexual privileges incorporated in that culture's sexual ideology and in the sexual scripts and erotica preferences of each gender.

P4   Social change and sexuality. For example: The institution that stresses flexibility the most will be the most likely to initiate change in other basic institutions. Therefore, since the economic institution is the most flexible, economic changes will be a key catalyst for changes in society.

The following paragraphs will comment on Reiss's theoretical perspective on science, his basic assumptions, aims, main societal features and propositions.

Scientific Perspective, Basic Assumptions

Reiss's work has been called holistic and Sprey (1988) notes that his 'strict adherence to positivist methodology are quite Durkheimian and solidly within the mainstream tradition'. Adams (1987) labelled Reiss's work as functionalist. The extracts of Reiss's propositions in the preceding sections bear out these descriptions to some extent, and Reiss's own views have evolved over time. In 1986b Reiss was convinced that an empirically-grounded science of the sexual could provide the means for Western society to understand and manage its sexuality in a rational and humane way. By 1993, however, he had reconsidered the meaning of the scientific basis of sexology. He now recognizes that sexual facts do not exist independently of the sexual science which explores them. Rather, that such science orders reality by making sense of it. This being so, the value of sexological theory must be made explicit at the outset. Reiss sees this in terms of reducing society's sexual problems. His insistence on making one's basic assumptions explicit is put into practice. Reiss (1993) exemplifies this issue when he compares the changes in the probability of HIV infection of two strategies (Reiss and Leik, 1989). He documents how colleagues with different presuppositions would interpret probability findings – with resulting different strategic recommendations.

Weaknesses and Strengths of Reiss's Premises

A number of the items considered by Reiss to be cultural universals can be questioned. Ethnocentrism and the expression of modern Western conceptions are perhaps most easily perceived through Reiss's commitment to self-disclosure. Gagnon (1987), for example, states, '. . . the very idea that sexuality should be a source of intimacy and emotional disclosure or that sexuality should be "other-directed" depends on a conception of the self . . . and the other . . . that is a singular product of the West.' Reflecting on the implications for clinical practice, Lavee (1991) argues that Western middle-class values tend to emphasize a) that sex is good, or at least natural, b) that sexual activity is on an interactional basis, and c) that partners should be equal in their relationships.

Similarly, Reiss had proposed to explain how cross-cultural differences in non-sexual patterns caused differences in sexual patterns. Udry (1986) argues, however, that he does not really maintain his cross-cultural purpose and is constantly wandering into areas where he feels biological explanations need to be established instead of describing the institutional correlates of variations in cross-cultural sexual patterns. As a cross-cultural comparison it is at risk of being ahistorical. From a methodological point of view, social anthropologists can find Reiss's uncritical use of ethnographic reports disconcerting. The importance of interpreting, rather than analysing, cultures needs to be carefully considered.

Simon (1986) acknowledges that the acceptance of the reality and coercive powers of social life is fundamental to all sociological analysis. Reiss, however, risks overestimating the reality of social life, reifying the concept into an almost living organism. He remains indifferent to the vital processes through which societal imperatives are linked to equally vital human desires. Moreover, it is observed that societies are dealt with as if they were equivalent mechanical arrangements of interacting parts that can be mapped by clusters of variables (Gagnon, 1987).

Others have already expanded on the implications of Reiss's belated appreciation of the profound reactive effect of the emergent sexological sciences on their subjects. Weeks's (1985) historical account of sexological work spans from the Victorian classifiers of deviations to Kinsey's examination of the variation in sexual behaviours in the USA in the 1950s. He has observed how supposedly neutral scientific classifications of the varieties of sexual behaviours have been used by those observed in the cause of their own political self-awareness as special groups. Thus, just as sexologists isolated the homosexual identity in the nineteenth century, they have unwittingly provided what Reiss has called *sexual scripts* for other sexual subcultures such as paedophiles, sado-masochists, etc. Such is the constituting effect of social science on its objects:

> Sexology, in association with the law, medicine and psychiatry, might construct the definitions. But those thus defined have not passively accepted them. On the contrary, there is powerful evidence that the sexual subjects have taken and used the definitions for their own purposes (Weeks, 1985).

In his still-optimistic post-positivistic vision of sexology devoted to human improvement, Reiss (1993) continues to underestimate the unanticipated and uncontrollable consequences which may lead from sexological research informing social policy. These issues notwithstanding, a consideration of Reiss's theory applied to furthering our understanding of sexual behaviour related to the risks of HIV infection clarifies the value in his approach.

The Macrosociological Perspective and HIV Risk

As Reiss's (1986b) theory is a societal-level explanation of sexual behaviour, it does not, at face value, seem useful for framing focused small-scale research, although by drawing on social and anthropological data it certainly highlights the importance of carefully contextualizing research designs. While his propositions specify the major sources of the societal determinants of sexual customs, few of them really explain cross-cultural sexual variation. The assumption of a meaningful link between cultural values and specific behaviour is at risk when applied to larger and highly differentiated societies that often represent a variety of subcultural experiences. Yet this is both a weakness and a strength if HIV risk is understood not merely in its Western sexual behavioural context, but in a global context in which modern differentiated cultures and traditional cultures meet and mix. The macrosociological perspective that incorporates the concepts of kinship, ideology, power and social change encourages this focus on AIDS as a global phenomenon and HIV risk as a consequence of cultural contact.

In applying Reiss's perspective to HIV, we look at the two key characteristics he considered generic building blocks of important human relationships. The first is physical pleasure and the second is self-disclosure. Pleasure exchange or communication of affection through touching probably is not the major goal or meaning of sexual contact for members of all subcultures in Western society. However, the physical pleasure potential in sexual relationships tends to be underestimated in social science research. More attention could be paid to this dimension, considering its importance among different gender, sexual orientation, social class and/or ethnic groups. Besides, to what extent do other tactile and visual sensations provide equivalent pleasures?

To the extent that the dominant culture in Western countries continues to stress the genitals as an erotic zone, it remains more likely that penetrative sexual contacts will be preferred, especially by males. Are men who equate physical pleasure in sexual contact mostly with penetrative sex more at risk of HIV infection than those who attribute less prominence to it? Reiss's claim that self-disclosure is an essential part of sexual encounters also merits consideration. Does, for example, the expectation of experiencing an enjoyable altered state of mind inhibit rather than promote openness and honesty about one's sexual history?

The interrelatedness of power and gender needs careful consideration when relating Reiss's theories to HIV risk. Consider for example the position taken by MacKinnon (1987), to wit, 'In feminist terms, the fact that the male has power means that the interests of male sexuality construct what sexuality as such means, including the standard way it is allowed and recognized to be felt and expressed and experienced, in a way that determines women's biographies, including our sexual ones.' Reiss (1986b) asserts, '. . . a more formalized theory of social power would allow for more precise formulation and testing of [these types] of propositions relating power to sexuality'. Stressing the relevance of social power in structuring sexual customs and interactions remains rather fruitless without specifying how power or other social factors operate.

Reiss's analysis suggests different sexual goals for subgroups in society that have different sexual ideologies. In an egalitarian sexual ideology the major goals are physical pleasure and psychological disclosure. For the proponents of non-egalitarian ideology it is heterosexual coitus. Tiefer (1991) acknowledges that Reiss posits the central role of patriarchy in contemporary sexual problems. However, she objects to his position as being one of the positions taken by the many well-intentioned liberal analysts who feel that patriarchy can be equated with male domination.

Large, complex societies with ideological systems that represent the views of contending groups will result in different conceptions of sexual normality from those of the social units in traditional face-to-face cultures. How does the distribution of certain types of power impact on sexual contacts between heterosexual partners? Does the impact of power differ if the contact is casual or committed? To what extent does a certain definition of sexual normality have an impact on preventive HIV-prevention programmes?

Reiss (1989) returned to his macrosociological perspective to examine what are seen as key sexual problems in contemporary American society. Unprotected intercourse and rape are both seen as consequences of the male–female power distribution, the training of men to be aggressive, and the persistence of gender roles that define the male as sexual initiator, and the female role as establishing the sexual pace and limits. Power expressed in gender roles takes the form of restraining and condemning female sexuality more strongly than male.

The perceived sexual crisis of the 1990s, in the form of AIDS, acquaintance rapes, teenage pregnancies and father–daughter incest, is traced to an unwillingness (among power-holding adult parents) to confront the consequences of the sexual revolution of 1965–75..Despite the fact that well over 80 per cent of all recently married women have had premarital coitus, there are millions of US citizens who are afraid that advertising condoms on network TV might promote illicit sexuality. The relevance of gender inequality is displayed in the very fact that advertising an easily available spermicide such as monoxymol-9 is not even debated.

Most young people in the USA do not discuss the control of pregnancy and disease prior to first coitus, as neither their parents nor society in general have made available suitable sexual scripts for this to happen. For the most part parents will not accept the sexual reality their teenage children face, unlike the situations that prevail in some European countries such as Sweden or the Netherlands. This takes the form of the culture's unwillingness to offer any media education on condom use based on the argument that promoting condoms is tantamount to undermining the accepted and right kinship, ideological and power structures.

In another book, *An End to Shame: Shaping our Next Sexual Revolution*, Reiss and Reiss (1990) castigate leading authorities and public figures for offering the public unscientific and moralistic messages which fail to acknowledge the reality of mainstream sexual behaviour:

> I believe that the low personal value placed on sexuality not based
> on love is what pressures many people toward an erroneous conclu-
> sion. All these anti-condom writers have indicated their low opinion
> of friendship/pleasure types of sex and have stressed the importance
> they place on committed love relationships (Reiss and Reiss, 1990).

They castigate a society torn between a Victorian resistance to promoting
condom use and a pragmatic urge to resolve the AIDS crisis. The result is a
society beset by a self-destructive sexual ambivalence and the creation of a
breach through which HIV may spread. Their pleasure/self-disclosure-based
sexual script theory offers a better means of understanding American intran-
sigence than the assumption that the issue is one of ignorance of the facts
combined with a lack of moral will to remove the traditional sexual blinders.
As Gagnon (1990) explains it, script theory applied to sexuality involves a
rejection of the widely held view that the human condition is defined as an
inevitable struggle between (fixed) individual needs and cultural proscriptions.
Rather, scripts are involved in 'learning the meaning of internal states, organizing the sequences of specifically sexual acts, decoding novel situations,
and setting the limits on sexual responses'. The adult society Reiss and Reiss
rage against has in its time adopted the sexual scripts of previous generations
and adapted them to manage prevailing conditions – in this case, the emergence of the HIV threat.

It is possible to draw some conclusions from this work as part of an
attempt to account for the social response to AIDS and the groups most at
threat. First, it should not be underestimated how such scripts help resolve
psychological tensions and provide the means for social organization. In
Journey into Sexuality (Reiss, 1986b) we learn about the boundary-maintenance
function of marital jealousy as the basis of kinship and as a means of expression of power.

It is unfortunate that Reiss should restrict his description of the manifestation of power to control access to sexuality in terms of gender roles, for
it is surely the case that power is also expressed in terms of generational
access to sexuality. Adults gain access to sexuality as a source of pleasure as
a right that is denied the younger generation. However, the price adults pay
for this is the kinship regulation of this access, i.e., the traditions of marriage
or at least stable relationships defined by the prevailing moral code.

The younger generation is involved in the process of exploring possible
future stable relationships, forming trial partnerships through their court-
ing rituals. Liberalization of controls over youth and the emergence of their
own subcultures has added the potential of open access to sexuality as part
of this experimental phase. In accordance with Reiss's original formula, the
dynamics of *sexual jealousy* surely appears as one motive underlying the prohibitions adults impose on their young, resulting in the contradictions he
bemoans.[4]

The physical and interpersonal rewards which sexual relations can offer are known to wane and can be short-lived. At the very least the frequency of sexual activity will decrease with age. Reiss (1986b) states that the loss of sexual fulfilment is the fate of many adult relationships and he reminds us of the large number of anorgasmic women in conventional marriages. Adult prohibitions concerning condom use by the young in their experimental relationships in the face of the AIDS threat can be understood as a rather destructive and punitive expression of power that is stimulated to some extent by generational sexual jealousy in addition to the more familiar rational motives (such as protecting the immature).

Our point here is that such a public reaction to the AIDS threat is not simply a matter of self-delusion or stupidity, as Reiss implies when he implores policymakers, parents and educators to *see sense* and *permit* or *allow* other kinds of sexuality. Weeks (1992) argues that both homosexuals (through the AIDS–bathhouse promiscuity connection) and the young are seen as violating a dominant shared sexual script by their respective de-coupling of sex and intimacy. The presentation of morality as a solution to AIDS reveals the psychic dimension of a sexual script that is imposed on youth (and other outgroups such as homosexuals) to control them punitively through the threat of fatal disease (Meredith, 1989). This dynamic should be viewed as a powerful organizer of the scripts by which adults tend to perceive the young (and homosexuals) as wanton sexual beings.

Another application of Reiss's perspective to understanding HIV-related risk behaviour is that dominant sexual scripts are limited in number and largely suited to adult life situations. On the whole they are neither available nor suited to young people's situations or needs. In contrast, young people are more inclined towards those fantasy (though powerfully-presented) sexual scripts created by the mass media, which, if not totally macho, are highly permissive, risky and arousing. These are what might be termed more accurately *proto-scripts*, insofar as they are unreal, idealized possibilities that are quite inappropriate to many young people's real-life situations.

Just as Reiss argues that homosexual behaviour results from an inability or unwillingness to live in a narrow, prescribed male script, so the young are unable to conform to adult scripts, in view of their circumstances. Both must resort to what they can pick up from elsewhere, that is, their own communities and the mass media. Reiss (1986b) has noted that 'some (shared) sexual scripting applies only to subgroups in society. For instance, homosexual scripting in the USA is largely unknown outside the homosexual community.' This should not be taken to imply that complete homosexual scripts are available to younger novitiates. Rather, they are likely to be as ill-defined as those available to heterosexuals.

Weeks (1992) has noted that the modern lesbian and gay male identities have been created by this process of self-organization and self-making, continuously from at least the eighteenth century, although he adds, 'There has been no linear development of a singular homosexual sense of self.' Reiss and Reiss (1990) tend to call on adult power holders to offer rational solutions to the young. In reality, young people, in much the same way as the gay community, will tend to draw on sexual scripts available from their own subcultures to manage the perceived HIV threat, rather than make use of what is handed down from above. In so doing they are asserting their own rights to a 'sphere of the intimate' outside the often punitive policing and jurisdiction of parents or adult power holders. The incidence of teenage pregnancy in the USA graphically reveals the price to be paid by young people when they draw upon the media-inspired sexual scripts available to (and preferred by) them. Moreover, during adolescence the psychological reward in risk-taking for its own sake is high, particularly where this involves violating accepted sexual scripts.

Before drawing our conclusions, we must emphasize that, as a tangent of interactionist social theory, the script device *per se* is opposed to conventional normative social theory. The theatrical metaphor was used to show that in modern societies people step in and out of roles that offer temporary identities. Applied to the sexual sphere, this contrasts with conventional notions of sexual socialization, in which one unconsciously takes on the norms (behaviours and values) passed on by the community or society. As Gagnon (1990) reminds us, we are socialized first as audiences to our teachers of cultural scenarios, but as we are required to enact these scripts we must modify them to meet the demands of the concrete situations in which we find ourselves.

Scripting as a sociological concept is more in tune with rapidly changing, differentiated, pluralistic, fragmented Western culture, in which a global media competes with the traditional forces of socialization to convey available and acceptable behaviours. Sexual experimentation and recreational drug use are by-products of late twentieth century urban life. Script theory is both a product of and most productive in explaining the nature of this cultural context.

With reference to kinship, ideology and power, young men and women are hetero- and homosexual social actors who have increasingly equal access to economic and social power. Kinship forces are marginalized and ideology commercially driven. This has created a relatively rapid reaction to perceived HIV-risk in the form of condom use, particularly in homosexual networks, even though, as Reiss is aware, USA teenager ignorance remains a problem.

However, it would be a mistake to address HIV-risk solely in terms of the adopted sexual scripts and corresponding individual rationalities of members of developed societies. Such sociological myopia fails to recognize that HIV-risk and transmission is a global rather than American or European phenomenon. After intravenous drug use, the epidemiology of HIV transmission point to intercultural contacts through travel and immigration as being major risk factors.

The greater prevalence of heterosexual HIV transmission in African and now Asian societies contrasts with that in developed societies. Many, otherwise traditional, African and Asian cultures have long-standing sexual mores that are far more libertarian than those of the post-Christian West. Nevertheless, in developing countries, kinship has regulated and continues to regulate sexual contact through the importance placed on children and property. Yet, given the impact of the economic breakdown that has affected African countries over the last two decades, kinship has been weakened by economic impoverishment and the ensuing mobility and urban drift. What affect has this had on sexual patterns? AIDS has been particularly devastating in communities in which prostitution and male-driven free sexual relations have overwhelmed the cultural boundary-maintaining functions of kinship (Caldwell *et al.*, 1989). In contrast to kinship and power, sexual script theory has less explanatory value in accounting for HIV risk-management in communities in which economically independent men, as a rule, are able to buy the sexual favours of economically dependent – and socially powerless – young women. In the belief that they are less at risk of contracting HIV, males pursue ever younger women for relationships, the consequence of which will be earlier infection. Such men are considering the meaning of safe sex, however erroneously.

This diversion has been included to draw attention to the danger of examining HIV-risk ethnocentrically and in terms of the rationalizations of relatively educated, socially powerful youth. The macrosociological perspective of sexuality outlined by Reiss contains within it concepts necessary to understand sexual behaviour and HIV-risk in both modern and traditional cultures and therefore the points where they increasingly meet.

Notes

1 Brief accounts of his theory are provided in two articles (Reiss, 1986a, 1989).
2 Major sexual ideologies and their tenets (Reiss 1986b, Table 5.1, p. 123).

Nonegalitarian sexual ideology
1 Males are more competent than females in the exercise of power, and they should be dominant in the major social institutions.
2 Body-centred sexuality should be avoided by females.
3 Sexuality is a powerful emotion and one to be feared by females.
4 The major goal of sexual relationships for females is heterosexual coitus.

Egalitarian sexual ideology
1 Males and females are equally competent in the exercise of power, and they should be treated as equals in the major social institutions.
2 Although person-centred sexuality is preferable, body-centred sexuality is acceptable for both males and females.
3 Sexual emotions are manageable by both males and females.
4 The major sexual goals for both males and females are physical pleasure and psychological disclosure.

3   In five causal diagrams, Reiss presents empirical data based upon analysis of the Standard Sample. This constitutes a subset of the Ethnographic Atlas, providing a selection of 186 best-described non-industrialized cultures, and purchased from the Human Relations Area Files. Reiss spells out in detail the way he carefully selected and used these data. Other sources mostly provide empirical evidence for North America and information from general sociological theory that fit with his prior theoretical positions.

4   In the UK, for example, members of the medico-scientific community involved in AIDS prevention during 1993 have begun increasingly to challenge the WHO-proclaimed statistical projections of the previous decade that HIV poses a serious threat to heterosexuals. The lack of anticipated increase of HIV-infection among young or older British, non-intravenous drug-using heterosexuals has led to the claim that the enormous expense of public education on the AIDS risk has been totally misplaced and unnecessary. Moreover, it is argued that it has merely had the questionable effect of introducing pre-adolescent school children to a range of minority sexual practices (scripts?), such as anal intercourse, of which they would otherwise have been unaware (see J. Le Fanu, *The Times*, London, 7 May 1993).

References

APFELBAUM, B. (1992) 'Book review (Reiss, 1990)', *Archives of Sexual Behavaviour*, **21**, pp. 93–5. + REISS, I.L. (Letter to the Editor): pp. 495–7.

CALDWELL, J.C., CALDWELL, P. and QUIGGIN, P. (1989) 'The social context of AIDS in sub-saharan Africa', *Population and Development Review*, **15** (2), June, pp. 185–234.

CARRIER, J. and BOLTON, R. (1991) 'Anthropological perspectives on sexuality and HIV prevention', in BANCROFT, J. (Ed.) *Annual Review of Sex Research*, **2**, pp. 49–75.

CATANIA, J.A., CHITWOOD, D.D., COATES, T.J. and GIBSON, D.R. (1990) 'Methodological problems in Aids behavioural research: Influences on measurement error in participation bias in studies of sexual behaviour', *Psychological Bulletin*, **108** (3), pp. 339–62.

DAVENPORT, W.H. (1987) 'An anthropological approach', in GEER, J.H. and O'DONOHUE, W.T. (Eds) *Theories of Human Sexuality*, New York: Plenum Press, pp. 197–236.

DAVIS, D.L. and WHITTEN, R.G. (1987) 'The cross-cultural study of human sexuality', *Annual Review of Anthropology*, **16**, pp. 69–98.

DELAMATER, J. (1987) 'A sociological approach', in GEER, J.H. and O'DONOHUE, W.T. (Eds) *Theories of Human Sexuality*, New York: Plenum Press, pp. 237–55.

DOCKRELL, J. and JOFFE, H. (1992) 'Methodological issues involved in the study of young people and HIV/AIDS: A social-psychological view', *Health Education Research*, **7** (4), pp. 509–16.

GAGNON, J.H. (1990) 'The explicit and implicit use of the scripting perspective in sex research', *Annual Review of Sex Research*, **1**, pp. 1–43.

GEER, J.H. and O'DONOHUE, W.T. (1987) *Theories of Human Sexuality*, New York: Plenum Press.

KON, I.S. (1987) 'A sociocultural approach', in GEER, J.H. and O'DONOHUE, W.T. (Eds) *Theories of Human Sexuality*, New York: Plenum Press, pp. 257–86.

LAVEE (1991) 'Western and non-western human sexuality: Implications for clinical practice', *Journal of Sex and Marital Therapy*, **17**, pp. 203–13.

MACKINNON, C.A. (1987) 'A feminist/political approach', in GEER, J.H. and O'DONOHUE, W.T. (Eds) *Theories of Human Sexuality*, New York: Plenum Press, pp. 65–90.

MEREDITH, P. (1989) *Sex Education: Political issues in Britain and Europe*, London: Routledge.

REISS, I.L. (1982) 'Trouble in paradise: The current status of sexual science', *Journal of Sex Research*, **18** (2), pp. 97–113.

REISS, I.L. (1986a) 'A sociological journey into sexuality', *Journal of Marriage and Family*, **48**, pp. 233–42.

REISS, I.L. (1986b) *Journey into Sexuality: An Exploratory Voyage*, Englewood Cliffs, NJ: Prentice-Hall.

REISS, I.L. (1989) 'Society and sexuality: A sociological explanation', in McKINNEY, K. and SPRECHER, S. (Eds) *Sexuality in Close Relationships*, Hillsdale, NJ: Lawrence Erlbaum, pp. 3–29.

REISS, I.L. (1992) 'Response to Tiefer's commentary on the status of sex research', *Journal of Psychology and Human Sexuality*, **5** (3), pp. 77–80.

REISS, I.L. (1993) 'The future of sex research and the meaning of science', *Journal of Sex Research*, **30** (1), pp. 3–11.

REISS, I.L. and LEIK, R.L. (1989) 'Evaluating strategies to avoid AIDS: Number of partners vs. use of condoms', *Journal of Sex Research*, **26** (4), pp. 411–33.

REISS, I.L. and REISS H.M. (1990) *An End to Shame: Shaping our Next Sexual Revolution*, Buffalo, NY: Prometheus Books.

SPREY, J. (1988) 'Current theorizing on the family: An appraisal', *Journal of Marriage and Family*, **50**, pp. 875–90.

TIEFER, L. (1991) 'Commentary on the status of sex research: Feminism, sexuality and sexology', *Journal of Psychology and Human Sexuality*, **4** (3), pp. 5–42.

WEEKS, J. (1985) *Sexuality and its Discontents*, London: Routledge & Kegan Paul.

WEEKS, J. (1992) *Against Nature: Essays on History, Sexuality and Identity*, London: Rivers Oram Press.

Book Reviews of Reiss, I.L. (1986b) *Journey into Sexuality: An Exploratory Voyage*, Englewood Cliffs, NJ: Prentice-Hall.

ADAMS, B.D. (1987) *American Journal of Sociology*, **93**, pp. 744–8.

ADERIDDER, L. (1987) *Family Relations*, **36**, pp. 225–6.

Fred Deven and Philip Meredith

GAGNON, J.H. (1987) *Contemporary Sociology*, **16**, pp. 238–40.
McKINNEY, K. (1987) *Teaching Sociology*, **15**, pp. 342–3.
SIMON, W. (1986) *Journal of Sex and Marital Therapy*, **12**, pp. 330–3.
SMITH, M.C. (1988) *Journal of Nurse-Midwifery*, **33**, pp. 243–4.
UDRY, J.R. (1986) *Journal of Marriage and Family*, **48**, pp. 683–4.
WHITAM, F.L. (1990) *Archives of Sexual Behavior*, **19**, pp. 531–4.

Chapter 9

Rationality and Preventive Measures: The Ambivalence of the Social Discourse on AIDS

Gustavo Guizzardi, Renato Stella and Jean Remy

The Individual and the Health Belief Model

From the standpoint of social spread of AIDS phenomenon, current models are inadequate to address the overall problem of sexual behaviour related to risk of HIV infection and all the various factors that enter into play. A new interpretive theory that could adequately confront the issue should involve a two-pronged approach. The first is to identify the areas where the Health Belief Model (HBM) can be criticized and to correct them. The second is to make an empirical study in order to pinpoint any essential aspects of the ongoing processes (Peto, *et al.*, 1992).

A main criticism is the presumption that there is a linear and consequential relationship between knowledge and behaviour. Pollak states, 'once the Health Belief Model is no longer used for practical purposes (designing and evaluating health educational programmes) its explanatory power easily looks like a tautology' (Pollak, 1992, p. 34). In view of the advice contained in this quote, we feel it is advisable in the beginning to leave aside the practical purposes that may unduly influence the theoretical construction. These, however, will be taken up at the end of the process. Pollak also says, 'the most fundamental criticism of the HBM is that in a way this model is no different from the conventional axioms of expected utility theory which are based on the assumption of rational individuals acting to maximise risk-benefit cost-benefit ratios' (*ibid.*, p. 35). His remarks address the two essential concepts of individual action and rationality. He does not develop these points completely. We should thus like to analyse them more fully.

The notion of network, in our view, is missing. We say this on the basis of research summarized in the final section of this article. Indeed, the crucial importance of small group relationships has emerged from the attempt to address AIDS-related problems and to interpret the situation as regards broad guidelines for communication.

Two Rationalities

In speaking of rationality we shall refer to the concept of health to keep our analysis concise and remain in the area of interest to us. Pearce (1989) and Sontag (1988) discussed health in at least two different cognitive frames of reference, medical science and an individual's life history. In medical practice the underlying assumption is often that individuals are willing to make sacrifices and act rationally in order to live healthily as long as possible. To achieve this they may even ignore needs or renounce pleasures that are detrimental to their health. From the standpoint of an individual's life-history, however, health tends to refer more to a notion of quality of life. The subjective choices made to preserve and maintain health vary highly from one individual to another and often contradict health strategies proposed by medical science. Individuals, in fact, tend to adopt forms of adjustment or compromise in order to pursue pleasures or satisfy needs which may nevertheless partly transgress or reinterpret responsibilities abstractly imposed by medical discourse. Smokers, for example, may, in a logic totally coherent to them, decide to combine both quantity and quality of life by smoking light cigarettes instead of giving the habit up completely. Similarly, the obese will cheat on their diets on special social occasions, such as dinners with friends or parties. Likewise, what we call in this study the *falling in love effect* could be usefully employed to illustrate this mechanism; when confronted with the risk, however well-known, of HIV, the individual takes a stance that is far from rational or consistent with the perception of the risk.

The problem we are discussing is, in fact, tied to two different notions and two different types of rationality: that proposed by medical knowledge, which is abstract and considered to be universal, and a concrete, pragmatic rationality that has come about subjectively, worked out in small networks of social relationships. Despite their contradictory natures, both rationalities exist side-by-side in the same social framework. In fact, the opposition between two rationalities of medical versus subjective lies less in a difference in meaning than it does in the different logics that govern them. The abstract medical logic attempts to impose an order in which health is paramount, whereas the individual, subjective logic arranges itself and adapts the unruly dimension of pleasure to medical discourse in a compromise that is often inconsistent. The predominant behaviour sets emerging from studies in Italy appear to confirm this interpretation.

This is particularly obvious with AIDS, since no social agreement has been reached between these two types of logic, as normally occurs in other circumstances. In modern dietary practice, for instance, medical injunctions coincide to some extent with the collective processing of values. As a result, the ascetic sacrifice of subjective pleasure is linked with gaining an advantage such as looking younger or more seductive.

The Question of Desire and Pleasure

These two rationalities are not congruent and, in fact, differ quite substantially on the question of desire and pleasure. This is evident in the highly ambivalent way the media links pleasure to sexuality. On the one hand sexual pleasure is loudly touted and legitimized through a wide variety of channels. Literature, advertising, the cinema and the press offer a bountiful and diversified range of messages presenting sexual pleasure as an individual goal that each individual has the right, the duty even, to pursue. On the other hand, the collective discourse on AIDS conveyed by the media and inspired by the rationality of the medical field calls explicitly for limiting sexual pleasure or at least employing some sort of control through suggested rules for safer behaviour.

If we look at the models of preventive messages put forward with regard to HIV infection, we can see the inherent contradictions more clearly, for here pleasure is not mentioned explicitly, merely alluded to indirectly. It is presented as an abstract, aseptic and neutral subject. In a word, sex is *medicalized*. By dressing it in a technical cloak of rational health and hygiene norms aimed largely at the use of condoms, preventive information undercuts the notion of sexuality. Pleasure is censored and is not mentioned as part of the message. Pleasure thus becomes the unspoken irrational component, even though it is taken for granted as the motivation and the end at the very heart of standards governing sexual behaviour. Pleasure is referred to only in terms of regulations. In other words, HIV/AIDS prevention messages recommend, in the name of health, limiting or abstaining from pleasure or adapting it to the use of condoms. In the case of AIDS prevention, this contradiction is even more flagrant from the moment that the pursuit of the pleasure touted by the media is seen as a cause of death.

The social discourse concerning drug dependency also contains a similar omission and censorship of pleasure, albeit in a different context characterized by a strong collective disapproval. This is especially true for the use of heroin and other substances taken intravenously, where preventive messages (concerning either drug dependency or AIDS) stress the context of anxiety, squalor and death that surrounds the use of these substances without any hint of the search for pleasure that may lie behind. Drug addicts are thus depicted as individuals who are basically irrational, whose drug-dependent behaviour can be explained only by a self-destructive urge, with the ultimate fate being self-destruction itself. Taking drugs becomes a logical nonsense; again the AIDS-prevention discourse manages to ignore its underlying ambivalence by limiting itself to indicating practical rational hygiene, such as not sharing needles. Of course, drug addiction also has its own culture, albeit to a lesser extent. Rock music, legendary figures of the beat generation and the biographies of famous 'damned souls' tend to form a counter-culture in the face of the spectre of death by drugs that is presented by the media. Although the influences of the two groups are not immediately comparable, one has to admit that the advocates of drugs do channel the appreciable and pleasurable aspects of drug use.

A somewhat similar analysis should be made of attitudes to risk (Vineis, 1990; Beck, 1992; Douglas-Calvez, 1990; McKeganey and Barnard, 1992). One cannot assume that individual behaviour is based solely on eliminating, or at least minimizing, risk in a subjective cost-benefit ratio. Once again the divide between abstract rationality and individual reasonableness is presented as an implacable contradiction. Here, too, the media plays a role in maintaining the ambiguity of this relationship in its social discourse on risk. Consider for a moment how modern society presents the taking of risks, even extreme, in a positive light. Sporting achievements and fictional heroism both on television and in films all celebrate the courage of those who dare to take risks (King, 1993).

The Collective Dimension

Another fundamental point in our analysis is the weight of the collective dimension. The objections raised by Pollak concern not only the notion of the logic behind action (i.e., the maximizing utility), but also the notion of agent. As he puts it, 'being centred on the individual, the HBM neglects the dynamic social interactions that shape the behaviour' (Pollak, 1992, p. 35). Nevertheless, an analysis centred on the collective dimension cannot be made as long as the notion of social is understood merely as a multitude of individuals, even though they may be interacting. Nor is it enough to include the existence of cultural models if they are taken merely as a common framework for the actions of several individuals.

Social Agents

A number of social agents act as collective agents with their own specific strategies, points of view, interests and networks of relationships. The main agents are those who are responsible for prevention information and campaigns (whom we shall call *preventers*), the recipients of the messages on health produced by the first group, the legitimate agencies for the production and elaboration of scientific research, and, last, the mass media.

It is interesting to note how the preventers are relatively ignored and their existence taken for granted. The overall assumption is that their social organization has no influence on the overall phenomenon and (for a large part) they are not conditioned by the collective dynamics of the social environment in which they operate. The existence of a feedback mechanism, whereby the preventers analyse the results of prevention campaigns as scientifically as possible and then modify them in accordance with the degree of success that they have assessed, measuring success in terms of the informative, communication or behavioural effects on the intended recipients, is generally accepted. This means that the originators of the messages are not considered to be part of the collective dynamics of communication.

The mechanism chosen is quite similar to that of a laboratory analysis in which

- the action complies strictly with experimental method, from identification of the problem to development of a stimulus to evaluation of the response and development of a new stimulus;
- society itself is the experimental field and is seen as the metaphor of a scientific laboratory;
- the experimenter is not considered to be part of the experiment.

We do not intend to analyse this view extensively; its limitations are clear to the preventers most aware of the problem. For example, there are occasions when the analysis of preventive campaigns leads them to stress the constant presence of one or another inter-experimental factor. Such a presence is often described as political (Wellings, 1992), although in reality it arises from more complex collective social factors.

A final key point is the role assigned to the legitimate agents involved in scientific research. Indeed, the assumption is they are also invested with the legitimacy to draw up social norms and propose ethical modes of behaviour. Thus, at the heart of the HBM lies a sociological problem in its strictest sense. The model's *knowledge–belief–behaviour* chain is not only problematic at its very core, which we can call the individual's rationality. It also runs into serious difficulties from the collective agent standpoint because agents are excluded from the analysis, albeit implicitly. The medical field, which in fact participates in the knowledge link of the chain, is placed outside the model when in reality it originated the model in the first place.

The complete model as seen by the preventers is actually as follows: The medical field develops knowledge and the non-medical recipients (individual or collective) adopt a behaviour in line with this knowledge. The link between them is the knowledge of the first group transposed into social norms and behaviour by the second. The sociological problem is how the transformation is understood. The aim, however, is not so much to understand how a correct transformation may be brought about (this is a problem for the medical field), but whether the fundamental process is characterized by the concept of transformation (Shinn and Whitley, 1985).

One should remember, however, that such an analysis is particularly difficult, given the peculiar characteristics of the HIV phenomenon. This is due to a series of factors that have shifted attention outside the medical field, placing the central role on individual behaviour. In fact, whereas scientific research appears to be capable of providing us with sufficiently thorough and reliable knowledge, at the same time it has a hard time using that knowledge to develop useful applications, whether for the treatment of those who have already contracted the disease or medical discoveries to protect the healthy (Mendes and De Busscher, 1993). Furthermore, this same scientific knowledge widened the gap between research and its useful application when it widely reported the extreme gravity of the phenomenon and its quite rapid spread.

Treating the disease has proved to be both socially and economically costly for society and, given the virus's global spread and long incubation period, these costs are likely to increase. As a result, society is giving less credence to the role and importance of the medical field precisely at a time when medicine is called upon to assume an even greater role. Hence there is the shift towards the perimeter to which we referred. Prevention through *treatment* is transformed into prevention through *information*, involving not only those who have contracted the disease or are particularly at risk, but the general healthy population as well. As a result, messages pertaining to the medical field evolve into ones that more aptly may be called social morality.

Short-circuiting Prevention

Prevention is the seemingly neutral term for the above-mentioned transformation of knowledge into behaviour. Collective communication is the main action within this process. In line with the overall mechanism, this communication contains two facets. The first – the seriousness of the collective problem – is general and descriptive; the second – the need for the population to change its behavioural patterns – is specific and prescriptive. The recommended behaviour changes, however, are by no means neutral, although they are often treated as if they were.

Treichler quotes the following statement as a paradigm of the present situation:

> Naturally we all know that the ultimate solution will eventually come
> to light in a laboratory. But meanwhile, what can the virologist or

microbiologist offer an AIDS victim and his or her loved ones to ease
their burden? To help them combat the ignorance and intolerance
they face which are growing day by day? (Treichler, 1992: 66)

This statement comes from a clearly prestigious official source: Dr Morisett,
Chair of the Programme Committee of the Fifth International Conference
on AIDS. The point is that something far from obvious has been taken for
granted, namely, that the virologist or microbiologist is legitimately required
to provide moral and ethical solutions, based on individual life-styles, for the
tragedy striking the sick.

The logical short circuit arises from the transfer of biomedical knowledge to the resolution of human dramas, whereas the sociological short
circuit arises from the transfer of the biologist's or doctor's legitimation from
a strictly experimental scientific field (the *laboratory* to use the earlier metaphor) to the social field. Why should a scientist who admits he cannot provide adequate scientific and medical means to fight the disease be seen as a
legitimation source to provide advice on behaviour, that is, in a field that is
not his own?

Treichler offers a close analysis of how this shift takes place, and how
the conflict within the biomedical field is gradually resolved by constructing
hegemonic positions for some groups. Treichler notes that 'a high degree of
correspondence is assumed between reality and biomedical models' (1992,
p. 68). This supports Kleinman's observation that 'the entry of the social
sciences into medicine has for the most part prompted not dialogue, but
an enriched biomedical monologue' (Kleinman, 1985, p. 75). Taussig adds
that the strange alliance between medicine and the social sciences has meant
that 'the issue is not the cultural construction of clinical reality, but the
clinical construction of culture' (Taussig, 1980, p. 12).

These considerations reveal a sort of vicious circle in the communication of prevention: If one is convinced that the knowledge–belief–behaviour
course is rational, then all unenvisioned or undesired behaviour patterns are
seen as deviations to be corrected. This means that prevention agencies
become further involved in the development and spread of norms once it
becomes apparent that the rules proposed by them have not been followed.
In fact, if one holds, for example, that irrationality can be imputed to ignorance, then preventers need only to increase the doses of rationality admin-
istered through informative communication. They are not aware, however,
that the error lies in mixing the medical-scientific sphere with the socio-
cultural sphere, or, rather, in believing that these spheres are contiguous when
they are actually two 'finite provinces of meaning' (Schutz, 1971, p. 206).

If we return to Morisett's quote, helping to combat ignorance has nothing to do with helping to combat intolerance. The first action draws its meaning from scientific procedure, where ignorance is contrary to knowledge.
Accordingly, an increase in knowledge will lead directly to a corresponding
decrease in ignorance. In the socio-cultural field, however, the opposite of

intolerance is simply tolerance; there is no direct cause-and-effect relationship between knowledge–ignorance on the one hand and tolerance–intolerance on the other. Increased knowledge may even be accompanied by increased intolerance.

The Multitude of Social Agents

The answer to our question about the strange transfer of legitimation from the laboratory to society – from scientific research to the issuance of precepts for daily life – is to be found in authority relationships and in the general process of developing collective norms of conduct.

In a macro-social collective arena behaviour and symbols and, above all, consensus are negotiated and interchanged in an often implicit process that is part of the dynamics of daily life. This dynamic process, best described as one of transaction–negotiation, is quite different from explicit dealings that occur mainly at set times and in set places (Perrinjaquet and Voyé, 1992). This transaction–negotiation process does not arise out of mutual concessions about norms that are imposed from outside (Remy, 1992). In the transaction, each participant contributes to an interactive process of defining the situation and building norms that culminates in a consensus on common values.

In the case of the HIV infection, the relationship is not merely between experts and 'normal people' (Roqueplo, 1974); the negotiation process also involves several collective agents. One agent is the organizations responsible for public health within the Welfare State (local authorities, town councils, public institutions, etc.). Another is the complex of political decision makers, who set broad policy guidelines by establishing budgets and allocating sizeable amounts of money and resources required to deal with the social emergency of the HIV infection (Scitovsky, 1989). A third is the world of technicians and experts (legal consultants, communications experts, economists, insurance agencies, bio-ethics scholars, etc.) who make an important contribution to the decision-making process. Last but not least, there are those who control symbols, for example, the church and other religious institutions.

These various agents interact in a complex network of mutual relationships where they are both overlapping and highly differentiated. It is a non-linear network, the most important characteristic being that it is not founded on an equal status in discourse, action and decision-making. We do not intend to go into this aspect here. Suffice it to say that this network exists and all its members have some degree of normative power and authority. However, this does not mean that the behavioural prescriptions formulated by these social agents are applied by the individuals whose daily lives they are intended to regulate (Backer, Rogers and Sopory, 1992; Kreps, 1988).

In a complex society there is no guarantee that the norms coming from various agents will converge, nor for that matter that the authority enjoyed in one sector may extend to actions in another. If anything, the very opposite usually occurs. In the case of sexuality one must also allow for the Luhmannian paradox that arises from both the radical distinction between personal and non-personal relationships and the fact that collective norms exist alongside the idea of the individual as absolutely self-referential:

> What one is looking for in love, what one is looking for in intimate personal relationships, is most of all a means to validate one's description of oneself... But if at a social level, one's description of oneself is seen as the 'formation' of one's own individuality, then it is precisely that which is in need of social support. (Luhmann, 1984, p. 200)

The interpretative model we propose is therefore one that is essentially macro-social, in which the various social agents at least seem to have independent normative powers and are able to impose descriptions of reality and behavioural norms. In reality, however, they are all actually negotiating with each other from different positions of power to gain overall status within the system, which by its very nature is unstable and provisional. It makes no sense, therefore, to talk about distortions, ignorance, and non-reception of messages, unless, that is, one adopts the point of view of only one of these social agents. At the end of the day, in fact, we are not confronted with a situation in which knowledge is developed by one source to be applied by another in a certain sphere of activity, but rather with the actual construction of collective discourse. Furthermore, this collective discourse represents not only the point of view of each agent involved, but also the situation of the system relative to the overall transaction–negotiation processes.

This view makes it possible to introduce an analysis of the mass media not merely as channels of information, but also as the recipients of ambivalence and the builders of a negotiated discourse at the collective level. This occurs in a public communicative area (Habermas, 1962) in which each collective agent develops his or her own particular conception of the situation and translates it into action that objectifies a specific point of view.

The Mass Media System

The central role of information and its impact on the behaviour of individuals tend to cast doubt both on expectations of rationality and on the very functioning of mass media in a complex society. The media is expected to act as a link between the intentions of the doctors and preventers and the choices made effectively by individuals (Berridge, 1992; Karpf, 1988). The media, however, is not neutral, nor does it act merely as a communication channel. Quite the contrary, it participates in the information process not only as a symbolic political arena in which the interests of the various social actors (doctors, politicians, associations, churches, etc.) involved in setting AIDS policies congregate, but also as a social agent in its own right.

Here we have another crucial fact that involves the construction of AIDS as something real. Even before dealing with preventive information and thus the overall set of behaviour norms, the media establishes the disease's social visibility. Were it not for television, radio and the press, knowledge of AIDS and its effects would have been limited to medical circles and to those who had direct experience with the disease, that is, were either infected or close to someone who was infected. On the contrary, the media has increased awareness greatly; it has created an information environment that offers space not only for prevention campaigns and news on scientific progress or the personal experiences of the sick, but also for the reactions this sparks both in public opinion and in the actors involved. The social visibility of AIDS thus means at least two things:

- the production of a discourse, be it medical, political or biographical, that takes the disease as its subject and makes its existence clear and believable;
- the establishment, due to the disease's social visibility, of a code whereby AIDS can be discussed in the framework of each actor's specific capacity.

This last point can be explained using a semiotic-textual model (Eco and Fabbri, 1978) in which both the transmitter and the recipient of information must refer not only to a code but also to a set of acquired textual practices and experiences, that is, the previous preventive campaigns or the tangible forms of individual and group processing of the disease's cultural and symbolic meanings. They are needed not only to communicate, but also to understand or interpret any part of the collective discourse on AIDS, which in the media gradually becomes just one of an infinite number of the media's genres of discourse. All this means that rationality is taken out of the communication process. The message that is sent does not always correspond to the message received because a number of different transformation factors intervene between the transmitter's intentions and the recipient's interpretation (Scherer and Juanillo, 1992). Not the least of these are the media's parallel discourses on sexuality, pleasure, illness, risk and death, which condition how the meaning is understood.

In short, inside his message the preventer constructs a *simulacrum* (Bettetini, 1984) of himself and of his own public in a relationship that obeys the rules of communicational rationality, i.e., 'I'll tell you what can harm you and you'll act accordingly,' expecting the message to 'work that way' and have the desired persuasive effect. However, the real addressee may not recognize himself in these simulacra but decode the message according to his own images of them inspired by a different rationality linked to his own behavioural background and ways of interpreting texts. An example of such an interpretation process is the logical 'near/far' dichotomy that governs what we have termed the *complexity reduction model* in our study.

So, far from being a simple, linear channel for the transmission of messages developed elsewhere, the media creates the conditions that determine what is real and speakable about AIDS. Each new message is added to the previous ones, and this is partially what gives AIDS its meaning.

The Complexity of the Media System

Further confirmation of the non-linearity of the communication model that governs how data and news about AIDS (or many other facts linked to collective emergencies) are circulated in a complex society can be found in other structural factors, namely the role and functioning of the mass media system itself. This system is to be understood as a non-coordinated set of messages coming from several sources and presented contemporaneously within the same social space (Poster, 1990). This allows us to construct a premise to define two elements of uncertainty or irrationality in the communicative processes, namely, the complexity of the information and the messages' contradictory elements.

By complexity we mean that individuals are not exposed to a single type of message (such as an HIV prevention campaign) but receive information from several channels at the same time (newspapers, television, films, literature). Each media has its own form of expression, ranging from documentaries and reports to drama, each with its own form of impact and context. These messages can either respect or counteract the rational preventive contents, for example, by focusing on the dramatic or sensational aspects. This is particularly true of news articles and stories, which also form the bulk of the messages available to the public. The individual must then call on a subjective reaction in order to reconstitute a coherent message from all the fragments received (Van Dijk, 1988).

Any hope of a clear correspondence between information and behaviour is thus shaken by the multiplicity of media and variety of expressive codes. Although it is not possible to establish, except through empirical research, what effect a message has on an individual's decisions and behaviour, it is possible to establish beforehand that such decisions have to take account of a structurally disorganized context. Thus, regardless of the choices an individual makes, he or she must give some logical consistency to the choices by excluding, summing, or including all or part of the messages received. This means that the reprocessing of information is not merely a question of idiosyncrasy or an effect of the social factors (age, culture, life-style, etc.) that condition the recipient, but is also part of the individual's own strategy to reconstruct meaning 'contractually' (Ghiglione, 1988). In other words, the media system is structurally incomprehensible without the individual selection and reformulation referred to above. Far from producing an incorrect (i.e., non-rational) interpretation of the messages, these steps provide the only possible means to interpret it.

By contradictory we mean that messages are not straightforward, but often ambivalent, when placed side-by-side, since not only do they pass through various channels, but they may well also emanate from social actors with different interests and ideological frames of reference. A good example is the disagreement that pits strict Catholics against most doctors and health authorities regarding the ethical issues surrounding the implementation of AIDS-prevention strategies in everyday life. This contradiction can also be seen in the different parts of a message, given that the media system in a complex society comprises a variety of production codes, message transmitters (with different aims and interests), and channels, the efficacy and impact of which may not be compatible.

This polymorphism finds its way into the messages themselves. It becomes a possible production and interpretation practice that establishes the empirical conditions for the contradiction we are discussing (Kitzinger, 1993). The contradiction may sometimes reside in the relationships between text and image as governed by the rules of major, rather than minor, reciprocal ambiguity (Barthes, 1980) or else in the relationship between the semiotic relation and content (Watzlawick *et al.*, 1967). On other occasions it can play on the presuppositions behind a message versus the openness of the same message (Eco, 1962). Lastly, as mentioned above, it can arise from misinterpretations of the simulacra of communication (Bettetini, 1984).

Collective Emergencies

A further aspect of the complex media system that deserves consideration is the structural multiplicity of a message's possible meanings. In fact, a general characteristic of the media, regardless of the matter covered, is to produce an interpretation that differs from the preventers' rational expectations. This is even more glaringly obvious in the case of AIDS, which has the nature of a collective emergency (Drabek, 1986; Dynes, De Marchi and Pelanda, 1987; Walters, Wilkins and Walters, 1989). Although the AIDS epidemic differs from the more common natural catastrophes (floods, earthquakes and forest fires, for example), it nonetheless has considerable effects on the function and role assumed by the media (Lazar, 1993).

The first effect is general. It is the creation of a powerful additional source of authority within the source itself that can legitimately tell people how to cope with the emergency. Crozier's (1964) remarks about power arising from a doubt resolved are especially true when the emergency by definition shows the gravity of the problem and the absolute need to solve it. On the other hand, one could argue with Luhmann that the emergency situation is a case of maximum contingency, that is, a situation that requires information coming from an extremely authoritative source, the content of which must be greatly simplified.

The intersection of a complex system and the need for simplified messages that attempt to describe an emergency or organize reactions to it reveals another aspect of the conditions of rationality. For the transmitter–preventer, these conditions should characterize the information and determine the apparently irrational situations in which the recipient understands and uses the information. Here again the behavioural choice arises from a process that is already problematic and contradictory, even without taking subjective motivations into account.

Sociologists refer to a situation in which the media is unable to respond quickly and effectively to an emergency as an *information catastrophe*. The delayed onset of symptoms and non-visibility of AIDS put us in uncharted waters compared with traditional crises and lead one to conclude that an information catastrophe is more the norm than the exception when it comes to the media's handling of the issue (Guizzardi, 1989). Furthermore, we should bear in mind that this information catastrophe is compounded by a *cultural* catastrophe due to the collective defensive reactions of prejudice and hunting for scapegoats (Stella, 1987; Guizzardi, 1987).

Recognition of the permanent state of irrationality that exists inside both the system and the discourse arising from the mass of messages it circulates is a first step towards a reorientation of thinking. The question is not why there is not always an adequate (i.e., rational) behavioural response to the intentions and strategies behind the messages, but rather how one can expect rational consequences from a system of media and messages built on different logical structures.

Research Results

Research conducted by Guizzardi and Stella in Italy[1] gives at least partial empirical support to the foregoing discussion of theoretical concepts. An analysis of the interviews showed that most of the basic prevention information in the messages, such as how the infection is transmitted and suitable ways of avoiding infection, had been acquired. As concerns the subjective processing of information, the positions that emerged from the interviews seemed to converge on a central, albeit non-explicit, position underlying the attitudes we observed throughout the analysis, namely, 'Does the AIDS problem concern me or not?'

In dealing with this implicit question the interviewees appeared to offer various models or subjective strategies for processing the complex communication and individual perception of AIDS-related risks. The predominant models we observed can be described in the following typology:

The irrelevance-type is one extreme hypothesis. Some respondents gave the clear impression that they did not consider AIDS a problem relevant to themselves, at least until they were asked to express an opinion on the subject. From the various themes developed during the interview we could deduce both the absence of social situations where AIDS is discussed (it is not talked about in the family, with friends or with the partner) and no direct acquaintance with people infected with AIDS or the HIV virus. The problem seems to be perceived as something unconnected to the individual and outside his or her direct experience, although there is still a certain degree of interest and curiosity about information (especially televised) about the disease or sensational events linked to AIDS (like the illness or death of a famous actor). Individuals with this attitude have sufficient preventive knowledge about the disease and how it is transmitted.

The first point of note is the contradiction between technical knowledge about AIDS and the subjective perception of the non-relevance of the risk that should logically follow and which, at least, is the intended effect of televised spots on prevention. This model, however, apparently sheds some doubt on the logic of information, since *knowing about* preventive norms does not lead to thinking that they *concern me* and even less so that I will put the norms into practice.

The absolute relevance type is another extreme hypothesis, at the other end of the scale of subjective perception and definition of risk. Basically this attitude can be summed up as 'The disease is everywhere and there is no way to defend ourselves'. In this case adequate behaviour does not involve specific preventive conduct but consists in simply avoiding everything and everyone. This attitude is more closely linked to the messages transmitted by the media than is commonly thought, and revolves around the *visibility–invisibility* dichotomy. The disease is, in fact, visible (we know it exists) through the media, but only through the media, because its presence in everyday life cannot be identified by symptoms and signs.

The contradiction between the way the disease is clamorously announced and constructed in the media and the absence of empirical means to verify the infection in everyday experience is resolved by giving an absolute value to the reality represented by the media even in daily life. The resulting attitude towards infection is one of hyper-attention, to the point where the individual avoids contact with objects and people in even the most commonplace situations. Even when the individual knows that the virus cannot be transmitted by contact, the general uncertainty of the situation leads to over-defensive behaviour, avoiding even those situations that the media have declared safe. Sometimes the whole path is reversed and the attitude adopted is erroneously attributed to the messages received, for example, 'I heard an interview where someone said you should avoid people who are HIV-positive and not touch them.' Another aspect of misinterpretation was expressed by some interviewees who thought the infection spread quite rapidly. This perception of rapid spread can be only partially imputed to the media; it is more a question of a subjective transposition of the utter gravity of the situation and the impossibility of coping with it.

A second major consequence of this contradiction in the media is that the individual does not hear the practical content of preventive information. The absolute importance given to the disease's threatening media visibility cancels out any of the messages' positive recommendations (using condoms, avoiding casual sex, etc.). Admittedly, this mechanism can be reinforced in cultures that stress the threatening aspects and oppose or discredit practical solutions. One example is the conflict between ultra-strict Catholics and the predominant pragmatic medical culture that lays the groundwork for official preventive norms.

The complexity reduction type is the central and most widespread type to emerge from our study. In this type the problem of the perceived risk is resolved by setting a boundary, a barrier of sorts, between the interpersonal reality of the individual's own social group and the world beyond. The 'real' risk is perceived as residing in the latter, i.e., the outside world, but not in the groups. This mechanism can be explained by the near/far dichotomy, which revolves around at least four basic hypotheses:

H1: By means of a collective, all-encompassing definition, the interviewees situate themselves spatially, almost geographically, in relation to the overall AIDS phenomenon. The most frequent perception under this first observation is that AIDS is primarily an urban phenomenon. Young people living in small towns, for example, tend to consider that AIDS occurs in the cities they are studying in, but not in their home towns. Those who live in the city regard it as closer to them but also restricted to another area.

H2: Another subjective defence mechanism lies in the circle of friends. In this case the attitude can be summed up as, 'Because I know the people I hang around with well, they are not infected.' In reality this mechanism is not as rational as it sounds, nor is it the result of any strict empirical examination. It can often be reduced to a circular argument along the lines of, 'My friends cannot be infected simply because they are my friends, just like I'm not infected because my friends aren't.'

H3: We have also found a perspective that is more specifically social or class-related (in the Weberian sense). Here a distant risk is attributed to a social category whose culture, educational level, habits, life-styles and the company they keep are different from the interviewee's. Once again the individual's own group is excluded from the risk, which is attributed to others.

H4: Another hypothesis revolving around the near/far mechanism is based on sexual distinctions. The most obvious case is that of the young women interviewed who saw AIDS as a sort of onslaught from the world of men that was about to be unleashed on them as well. A distant phenomenon was closing in. This perception is partly linked to the history of the epidemic, which was first reported in male homosexual populations, then spread among the heterosexual population. However, for the young women interviewed, the notion of heterosexual in the context of AIDS merely reinforced the idea that the infection came from the other sex, in other words, quite simply from men.

In Italy this is an especially crucial factor, since from the very beginning the disease was observed to be transmitted primarily not by homosexual contact, but by drug addiction. The link between AIDS and drug addiction is certainly related to sharing needles, but also to sexual relations between infected drug addicts and the general population. This emphasis on the purely (or at least predominantly) sexual route of infection and the related risk is thus an important factor that merits further research.

One might well think that the above attitude concerns a couple, that is a man and woman in a stable relationship who have sexual relations. We have seen, however, that this generally is not the case. On the contrary, the near/far type is the most prevalent. Young couples tend to avoid discussion of AIDS, rarely mention it explicitly, and do not check whether there is any real risk of AIDS. Instead, they tend to follow the illusory *knowledge* criteria (another form of *near*), that is, 'I know who my partner is and I am aware of his or her past history, so this makes me safe.'

Types in Crisis

This typology of those who see AIDS as irrelevant, completely relevant, or attempt to reduce complexity, defines and tests attitudes towards the HIV risk but nevertheless does not entirely explain the interviewees' positions. Other elements, which, in fact, often constitute the very limits of the types themselves, are involved. The main ones are:

Comparisons with reality

The most basic example of this confrontation with reality occurs when an individual observes cases of infection (AIDS or HIV-positive) or persons highly at risk in his or her own reference group. The most prevalent reaction to such a situation is to retain, while adding to new elements to, the complexity reduction model. The first element is to erect another barrier, which we call *mental distancing*. When, for example, an interview brought out that the individual actually did know people diagnosed with AIDS or HIV carriers, including people in his or her proximity (classmates, neighbour, the landlord of a local pub), it was striking to see how these facts were recalled with difficulty, often only after the interviewer had insisted in the face of initial and occasionally repeated denials by the interviewee. The second element consists in shifting prior established boundaries and reducing the near area to a more restricted context. The distant which has become closer is once again pushed beyond the area of relevance. Examples of this reaction can be no longer seeing someone who is HIV-positive, or the group's ceasing to meet at the pub whose landlord has AIDS or is even suspected of having it, etc.

We can see the inherent limits to this mechanism in the way it is applied. The implicit message is that it is only temporarily valid; in the long run it is no longer sustainable. The model is based on the premise that, 'My group is invulnerable', which in the end proves unfounded. The devastating effects of the shaken premise are mitigated by redefining the group's boundaries and constricting the safe zone. At the same time, however, the individual must confront not only the evidence that the premise does not work, but also two messages conveyed by the media, namely, that no one is excluded from the risk of infection and suitable behaviour is not that of the safe *group* but that of safer *sex*. We should also mention that the model would be truly shaken when an individual learned that someone from his or her own or a close group had died of AIDS. We did not encounter enough cases in our study, however, to state this with certainty.

Necessary sexual otherness

Another limitation to the complexity reduction model is the fact that the safe group solution cannot be applied to sexuality. This is all the more true for males, for whom the near/far dichotomy partly assumes a more extreme aspect in the form of inside/outside. The underlying distancing mechanism is that AIDS is a disease of homosexual males. As the implicit affirmation is, 'I am not homosexual', we were thus told explicitly, 'I am not in the AIDS risk group; I am "outside" by definition.' Nonetheless, even though the interviewees were able to state their certainty of being HIV-negative themselves because of their own individual life histories, this does not mean they could be equally sure about a woman with whom they had sex, even though she belonged to the safe group. This is precisely what negates the validity of the safe group criteria, one of the key elements of the complexity reduction model.

The falling in love effect

A final, and extreme, limitation is what we call the *falling in love* effect, found mainly among the female respondents. The typical attitude is, 'Today I am not at risk, but someday I could become infected if I fall in love with an HIV-positive man and have sex with him.' The code of love is the most radical transgression of all rules of safety and prevails over any other model defining sexual risk. There is, in fact, a wide gap between, 'I must change my attitude' and 'I will surely change my attitude', found mainly among the women interviewed. Moreover, women have a greater tendency than men to grasp the wide discrepancy between knowing what safe conduct should be and actually putting the acquired knowledge into action, especially with a man to whom they are attracted.

Conclusions

It is our view that in a complex society the only realistic objective preventers can hope to achieve is to maximize the effects of their intervention, given that the starting conditions are often unknown, ill-known or distorted. On the question of communication, it is useful to distinguish between two levels, namely, mass communication and other levels of communication that target more restricted groups.

At the mass communication level we must realize that the most easily attained objective is almost solely that of informing the public. We should thus abandon the notion that general changes in behaviour can be induced by the mass media. This is confirmed by the results of recent mass communication research (Atkin and Wallack, 1990; McQuail, 1987; Wolf, 1985) showing that it is time to renounce any claims about the power of the media and adopt a more realistic micro-physical view of their ability to influence.

Instead of defining key solutions on behaviour to impose on the target population, we really need targeted research to identify the key actors – the social interface between the public sphere and the network of interrelations so important for specific groups. There is an even greater need to identify and conduct in-depth studies aimed at developing a typology of network relationships, as the latter are known to be crucial strategic arenas for developing attitudes and in part the responses – even individual responses – to the problem of AIDS. This implies less emphasis on epidemiological distinctions between high-risk groups and behaviours. These distinctions are based on statistical probability hypotheses which, although possibly helpful in explaining certain aspects of the phenomenon, are relatively useless, if not dangerous, in the operative field, where the goal is to limit the spread and effects of AIDS.

We know that the AIDS phenomenon involves at least three relational levels, namely, intimate, interpersonal group and the macro-collective, and that specific interpretations, attitudes and behaviours are developed at each of these levels. We should also realize that preventive actions should never confuse the three levels. Above all, we should refrain from attempts to transfer the mechanisms valid for one level to others. We must avoid the error of thinking that the authority held by specific agencies at the macro-social level is automatically transferable to the other relational levels. More specifically, the conditions of a collective emergency, which appear so obvious macro-socially, carry much less importance at the other two levels and do not seem to be capable of producing the same types of interpretation of the AIDS phenomenon.

Returning to what we said earlier with regard to communication, we should consider actions combining the different levels of communication (media, groups and networks, and face-to-face) in a mixture of initiatives that establishes the conditions for complementary, mutually reinforcing messages. We should also take into account the findings of social marketing research (Tamborini, 1992).

Note

1   The research was conducted on a sample of 157 young people of both sexes, between the ages of 19 and 24. Each individual was interviewed in depth. The research was funded by grants from MURST and CNR in Italy.

References

ATKIN, C. and WALLACK, L. (Eds) (1990) *Mass Communication and Public Health: Complexities and Conflicts*, London: Sage.

BACKER, T.E., ROGERS, E.M. and SOPORY, P. (1992) *Designing Health Communication Campaigns: What Works?*, London: Sage.

BERRIDGE, V. (1992) 'AIDS, the media and health policy', in AGGLETON, P., DAVIES, P. and HART, G. (Eds) *AIDS: Rights, Risk and Reason*, London: Falmer Press, pp. 13–27.

BARTHES, R. (1980) *La chambre claire. Note sur la photographie*, Paris: Gallimard-Seuil.

BECK, L. (1992) *Risk Society, Towards a New Modernity*, London: Sage.

BETTETINI, G. (1984) *La conversazione audiovisiva*, Milano: Bompiani.

BLANC, M. (Ed.) (1992) *Pour une sociologie de la transaction sociale*, Paris: L'Harmattan.

COSTANZI, C. and LESMO, C. (Eds) (1991) *Adolescenti e prevenzione dell'Aids*, Milano: Angeli.

CROZIER, M. (1964) *Le phénomène bureaucratique* (trad. It. *Il fenomeno burocratico* [1970] Milano: Etas Kompass).

CROZIER, M. and FRIEDBERG, E. (1977) *L'acteur et le système. Les contraintes de l'action collective*, Paris: Seuil.

DICLEMENTE, R.J. (Ed.) (1992) *Adolescents and Aids*, London: Sage.

DOUGLAS, M. and CALVEZ, M. (1990) 'A self as risk-taker: A cultural theory of contagion in relation to AIDS', *Sociological Review*, **38** (3), pp. 445–64.

DRABEK, T.E. (1986) *Human System Responses to Disaster*, New York: Springer.

DYNES, R.R., DE MARCHI, B. and PELANDA, C. (1987) *Sociology of Disasters*, Milano: Angeli.

ECO, U. (1962) *Opera aperta*, Milano: Bompiani.

ECO, U. and FABBRI, P. (1978) 'Progetto di ricerca sull'utilizzazione dell'informazione ambientale', in *Problemi dell' Informazione*, **4**, pp. 127–44.

GHIGLIONE, R. (1988) *La comunicazione è un contratto*, Napoli: Liguori.

GUIZZARDI, G. (1987) 'Chernobyl. L'esplosione dei media', *Politica ed Economia*, **6**, pp. 49–56.

GUIZZARDI, G. (1989) 'Il fenomeno Aids tra catastrofre informativa ed esosrcismo tramite comunicazione', in CRESPI, F. *Sociologia e cultura*, Milano: Angeli, pp. 369–77.

HABERMAS, J. (1962) *Strukturwandel der Oeffentichkeit*, Luchterhand, Neuwied: Verlag.

KARPF, A. (1988) *Doctoring the Media: The Reporting of Health and Medicine*, London: Routledge.

KING, S. (1993) 'The politics of the body and the body politic: Magic Johnson and the ideology of AIDS', *Sociology of Sport Journal*, **10** (3), pp. 270–85.

KITZINGER, J. (1993) 'Understanding AIDS: Media messages and what people know about acquired immune deficiency syndrome', in Glasgow University Media Group (Eds), *Getting the Message*, London: Routledge.

KLEINMAN, A. (1985) Introduction to GAINES, A.D. and HAHN, R. (Eds) *Physicians of Western Medicine: Anthropological Approaches to Theory and Practice*, Dordrecht: Reidel.

KREPS, G.L. (1988) 'The pervasive role of information in care and health care: Implications for health communication policy', *Communication Yearbook*, **11**, pp. 238–76.

LAZAR, J. (1993) 'Les medias et les rumeurs en temps de crise: Analyse de divers discours sur le sida', *Communication-Information*, **14** (1), pp. 129–46.

LUHMANN, N. (1984) Soziale Systeme, Frankfurt: Suhrkamp, Verlag (trad. It. *Sistemi Sociali* [1990] Bologna: Il Mulino).

LUHMANN, N. (1982) *Liebe als Passion. Zur Codierung von Intimität*, Frankfurt: Suhrkamp, Verlag.

MCKEGANEY, N. and BARNARD, M. (1992) *AIDS, Drugs and Sexual Risk*, Buckingham: Open University Press.

MCQUAIL, D. (1987) *Mass Communication Theory: An Introduction*, London: Sage (trad. It. *Le comunicazioni di massa* [1993] Bologna: Il Mulino).

MENDES, L. and DE BUSSCHER, P.O. (1993) 'Un Bouleversement scientifique? Les Sciences humaines et sociales face a l'epidemie du sida', *Sociétés*, **42**, pp. 351–6.

MORISSET, R.A. (1989) 'Abstracts and program', presentation at the Fifth International Conference on AIDS, International Development Research Centre: Montreal, Ottawa.

PEARCE, B.W. (1989) *Communication and the Human Condition*, Southern Illinois University Press.

PERRINJAQUET, R. and VOYÉ, D. (1992) 'Nouvelles frontières médiatiques, nouveaux espaces sociaux', *Espaces et Sociétés*, **50**, pp. 175–94.

PETO, D., REMY, J., VAN CAMPENHOUDT, L. and HUBERT, M. (1992) *Sida. L'amour face à la peur*, Paris: L'Harmattan.

POSTER, M. (1990) *The Mode of Information*, Cambridge: Polity Press.

POLLAK, M. (1992) 'Attitudes, beliefs and opinions', in POLLAK, M., PAICHELER, G. and PIERRET, J. (Eds) *AIDS: A Problem for Sociological Research*, London: Sage.

REMY, J. (1992) 'La vie quotidienne et les transactions sociales: Perspectives micro ou macro-quotidiennes', in M. BLANC (Ed.) *Pour une sociologie de la transaction sociale*, Paris: l'Harmattan, pp. 83–112.

ROQUEPLO, PH. (1974) *Le partage du savoir: science, culture, vulgarisation*, Paris: Seuil.

SCHERER, C.W. and JUANILLO, N.K. (1992) 'Bridging theory and praxis: Reexamining public health communication', *Communication Yearbook*, **15**, pp. 312–45.

SCHUTZ, A. (1971) *Collective Papers*, The Hague: Nijhoff (trad. It. *Scritti sociologici* [1976] Torino: Utet).

SCITOVSKY, A. (1989) 'Studying the cost of HIV-related illnesses: Rflections on the moving target', *Milbank Quarterly*, **67** (2), pp. 318–544.

SHINN, T. and WHITLEY, R. (Eds) (1985) *Expository Science: Forms and Functions of Popularisation*, Dordrecht: D. Reidel.

SONTAG, S. (1988) *AIDS and its Metaphors*, New York: Farrar, Straus and Giroux.

STELLA, R. (1987) 'L'epidemia da Aids come disastro culturale', *Inchiesta*, **75–6**, pp. 86–93.

TAMBORINI, S. (1992) *Marketing e comunicazione sociale*, Milano: Lupetti.

TAUSSIG, M.T. (1980) 'Reification and the consciousness of the patient', *Social Sciences and Medicine*, **14B**, pp. 3–13.

TREICHLER, P.A. (1992) 'AIDS, HIV, and the cultural construction of reality', in HERDT, G. and LINDENBAUM, S. (Eds) *The Time of AIDS*, London: Sage.

VAN DIJK, T.A. (1988) *News as Discourse*, Hillsdale: Erlbaum.

VINEIS, P. (1990) *Modelli di rischio: Epidemiologia e causalità*, Torino: Einaudi.

WALDBY, C., KIPPAX, S. and CRAWFORD, J. (1993) 'Heterosexual men and "safe sex" practice', *Sociology of Health and Illness*, **15** (2), pp. 246–56.

Gustavo Guizzardi, Renato Stella and Jean Remy

WALTERS, L., WILKINS, L. and WALTERS, T. (Eds) (1989) *Bad Tidings: Communication and Catastrophe*, Hillsdale, NJ: Erlbaum.

WATZLAWICK, P., HELMICK BEAVIN, J. and JACKSON, D. (1967) *Pragmatic of Human Communication: A Study of Interactional Patterns, Pathologies, and Paradoxes*, New York: Norton.

WELLINGS, K. (1992) 'Assessing AIDS prevention in the general population', *Cahiers de Recherche et de Documentation*, Lausanne: Institut universitaire de médicine sociale et préventive.

WOLF, M. (1985) *Teorie delle comunicazioni di massa*, Milano: Bompiani.

Chapter 10

Operationalizing Theories for Further Research

Luc Van Campenhoudt

Progress has been made in the past few years in moving from individual-oriented to interactional-oriented perspectives for the purpose of explaining sexual behaviour related to the risk of HIV infection. The authors in this book have contributed to this effort and have noted the importance of the relationship, social networks and cultural and contextual influences on sexual behaviour. A number of recent investigations from which the contributors to this book have drawn inspiration show that these perspectives can be used in specific research to yield useful information about sexual behaviour. It might be possible to use them even more quickly, more often, and with better results under certain conditions that will be explored in this chapter.

Toward a Critical and Structured Eclecticism

The chapters in this book call attention to the extreme complexity of the sexual behaviour. It is characterized by the intertwining of personal, relational and socio-cultural aspects and involves all dimensions of the personality, i.e., intellectual, mental, emotional and physical. In spite of this complexity or, more to the point, because of it, we should abandon the belief that good research is possible only if it relies on sophisticated theoretical models that have been developed meticulously. Adding more elements to already complex models is unlikely to further the knowledge about why persons engage in different types of sexual activity. For example, when models like the HBM failed to explain sexual behaviour as a result of individual-oriented factors, adding more factors such as self-efficacy and locus of control did not prove to greatly increase their predictive power. Moreover, if a theory is not flexible enough, it will smother, rather than elucidate, phenomena. An experienced researcher will always go farther with just a few pertinent key questions and a good knowledge of recent research in the field than the researcher who wields, in a stereotyped manner, what Edgar Morin called *ignorant knowledge* (*savoirs ignares*), however sophisticated this ignorant knowledge may be.

Many contributors to this book stress the importance of not locking oneself into overly sophisticated theoretical frameworks. Instead, they give priority to a good description of the interaction processes under study in order to understand them fully. This means inverting the ratio between theory and method. According to this line of reasoning, the theory becomes a component of a method in the broad sense of the term. Theory and method become an integrated scheme for exploring reality. This does not mean denigrating the theoretical work. Instead, it provides the reference points and main axes of the research aimed at elucidating the issues and constantly recomposes itself as this work progresses. From such descriptive research one can extract scripts, sequences of interactions or typical scenarios that can be used to locate singular situations and understand better their underlying logic.

The corollary is the need to limit the ambitions of each research project, to limit both the scope of the study (for example, one type of population or situation, one dimension of the sexual relationship, and so on) and the theoretical and methodological approaches that are taken. No single theory will one day be able to explain validly, on its own, all of the phenomena under study. Sexual behaviour must be seen from a diversity of perspectives that are not necessarily compatible. All theories are contingent and must change with changes in their scopes. The diversity and limits of the approaches presented in this book are further proof of this. However, the theoretical eclecticism and flexibility that are advocated here should be anchored in a structured theoretical and scientific space. Otherwise, they lead to relativism and the shattering of the theoretical field. One must be able to identify each approach's epistemological foundations and the latter's implications, such as the type of empirical work that they require or the validity of the information that they yield.

In the discussion chapters as well as in the introductions of the first three parts, criteria have been proposed for situating each perspective in the theoretical space. Two distinctions have been proposed: the first is between formal and material causes, the second between different types of explanation or causality. Formal causes establish the rules for a theory and determine probabilities of outcome behaviour, while material causes provide insight into the actual circumstances leading to a particular behaviour (see Introduction to Section One). With regard to the second distinction, the main different types of explanation or causality are systemic, functional, actancial, dialectic and hermeneutic. Each perspective combines different types of explanation and gives a different weight to each of them. The social system theory approach (Ahlemeyer) combines systemic and functional explanations. The social network theory approach mostly obeys a systemic explanation, but Ferrand and Snijders envisage combining it with an actancial explanation. The cognitive and social psychology approach (Ludwig) combines actancial and hermeneutic explanations. The relational sociology approach (Bastard, *et al.*) relies mostly on an actancial explanation after considering the uselessness of hypotheses based on a linear causality. Deven and Meredith combine Reiss's anthropological approach, which relies on systemic and functional explanations, with an actancial perspective. The critical and constructivist sociology approach of Guizzardi, *et al.*, combines actancial, dialectic and hermeneutic explanations.

If we are aiming for a satisfactory and sufficiently broad explanation of sexual behaviour related to the risk of HIV infection, we must try to meet two requirements. First, we must include a formal and a material component in whatever explanation is chosen. Second, we must allow for the three complementary dimensions of human and social phenomena that are, according to Berthelot's terminology (1990), structure, process and meaning. Of course, it is not necessary or even possible to give the same weight to those different dimensions in all research systematically. This is why comparing and articulating research findings based on different perspectives is indispensable. This is what we tried to do in this book, from epistemological benchmarks aimed at clarifying the debates and avoiding misunderstandings. From this comparative point of view, the scope and limits of each approach can be better considered and one can see better what should be taken into account more.

To achieve theoretical progress, one must be able to consider research itself to be part of the subject matter under study, especially as a component of the collective process of constructing representations of the AIDS problem and its prevention, as Guizzardi, Stella and Remy have shown. Social scientists cannot legitimate their intervention by seeking to place themselves outside the bounds of a game in which they are perhaps increasingly important players. To paraphrase Pierre Bourdieu, the condition of sociological knowledge of a social phenomenon is a critical sociology of the sociological work on this phenomenon.

All the above conditions may be met only if one engages in a dialectically-motivated theoretical and meta-theoretical discussion (epistemology, sociological criticism of knowledge). The social scientist must constantly lay bare and try to overcome the contradictions that exist between theoretical approaches and research findings in order to build constantly emerging knowledge. We are not searching for a certain level of quality and quantity of knowledge defined as the ideal situation. On the contrary, we are trying, through conflictual co-operation, to give birth together to a knowledge process that has some significance with regard to the burning issue of AIDS. The ultimate criterion of science is nothing more than the inter-subjectivity of researchers.

Some Theoretical Issues

Under those conditions of clarification and discussions, it should become easier to build upon theoretical developments. For example, we have discerned four promising theoretical tracks in the discussions in the previous chapters. These tracks are described briefly below.

The first one concerns the non-hierachical vision of social reality which implicitly underlines several perspectives presented in this book. In order to explain sexual behaviour related to the risk of HIV infection, the social system is seen as a system of reciprocal, circular determination among cultures and macro-social processes, institutions and political and institutional processes (this level is not always separated from the previous one), the micro-social level of organizations, and the level of interpersonal relations. This non-hierarchized vision of the levels of social reality is at odds with the conventional vertical vision of the social system, where micro-social processes are produced by macro-social phenomena but do not produce the latter in return. It also contrasts with an asocial view of relations in which actual relations are considered in isolation from their macro-social contexts. The study of sexual relations' connections with the other levels of social reality thus does not consist in analysing how the sexual relationship is determined by contextual dimensions that are external to it.

On the contrary, it means studying how, inside their relationship, the partners come to grips with the elements of the context that are deemed to be both constraints and resources that set the boundaries of a more or less broad set of possibilities. The major implication of this point of view for research is that interactions must be considered a (and doubtless *the*) key subject of analysis, for they have a decisive role in determining the partners' behaviour and meanings.

A second promising track is the importance given to social micro-networks in determining effective sexual norms. These networks are viewed as the conceptual bridge between macro-social processes and the partners' relationship. The partners' effective norms and behaviour patterns crystallize primarily at this level. The authors in this book who have covered the subject explicitly consider these micro-networks to be systems of interactions. Still, examining them will not reveal the course that the relationship will actually take. In other words, they determine a probabilistic framework only.

A third promising track is the insistence on the relative autonomy of intimate systems. The sexual relationship has its own dynamics. It is a relatively autonomous system in that it consists of a process of mutual behavioural adjustments designed to allow the relationship to develop in a way that is acceptable to both partners. The relationship is thus self-referential. In these processes of transactions between partners and mutual adjustment, each partner's behaviour is also driven by the desire to reinforce a certain self-image, to pursue one's own aims, to rule out certain worries. The degree to which the relationship is open or closed to its social environment may not be studied independently of the relationship's internal demands and those of the partners.

A last track explored in this book is the idea that the partners' interactive behaviours and meanings are the building blocks of the relationship. A relationship-oriented approach takes into account the partners' interactive behaviour and meanings rather than the individuals' own characteristics. By interactive behaviour and meanings we mean what constitutes the relationship and has significance only with respect to the relationship and the other partner, for example, dominating and submissive behaviour in line with the partners' respective resources, mutual rapprochement or avoidance behaviour, verbal exchanges, and everything through which they express their images of this relationship (such as proposing or not proposing to use a condom), their desires and expectations, and, above all, the meaning the relationship has for each of them. These interactive behaviours and meanings are forms of communication.

The relationship is a set of interactive behaviours and meanings that gives it life and substance. In an interaction-oriented approach these interactive behaviours and meanings are incomprehensible if they are considered separately from each other. They are elements or moments in connected sets of interactions that are called systems or sequences of interactions, depending on the theoretical perspective that is adopted and whether one favours a structural or dynamic explanation. Analysing the sexual relationship then boils down to revealing the structures and/or chains of interactions. If the aim of research is to explain specific behaviour, such as proposing or refusing to use a condom, this behaviour should be considered not the effect of the relationship, but a component of the relationship that is consequently explained by its position in a structure (or a system) and/or a sequence.

Such a perspective does not necessarily overlook or underestimate contextual elements and individual characteristics; it recomposes them in line with the relationship's structural or dynamic logic. Thus, a macho male will adopt macho behaviour even more frequently if his partner submits to such behaviour or even asks for it implicitly; one of the partners will rely even more on the resources of his or her education if the couple finds itself speaking about AIDS extensively and often; the involvement (for example, matrimonial or romantic involvement) of each of the partners will be reinforced or weakened by the other partner's responses, etc. If we subscribe to these theoretical considerations, we must deduce from them some specific methodological consequences.

Which Methods (in the Narrow Sense) for the Subject?

If the sexual relationship is the chief subject of analysis and its components are the interactions between partners, then the researcher's main task is to understand how these interactions unfold and to elucidate the links between them, the processual and the structural logic, and the meanings that underlie them. In the final analysis, that is where risks are or are not taken, the influences of the social environment and cultural context are felt, social roles are acted out with more or less conformity, effective norms are renewed or transgressed, and the relationship's meaning crystallizes and re-crystallizes with the march of time and events.

We have underlined both the semi-randomness and singularity of these interactions. In one corner we have structures, systemic logic, scripts, behaviour patterns and power structures. In the other corner we have the irreducible singularity and self-referential nature of each individual and each relationship, the contradictions that are resolved in the unexpected, the unforeseen event or circumstance and the specific meaning that each individual gives to his or her own experiences. The texts in this book propose various reference points and/or types of conceptualization to help plot one's course in the study of such a subject. Some of them may be referred to by their corresponding key words, to wit, intimate systems, transactions and negotiations, bargaining, phases of the relationship and sexual scripts.

We have seen that each approach forms a whole, that the theory cannot be separated from the methods, especially if the theory is construed to be a component of the methods, themselves understood in the broad sense of the term. We have also seen that the empirical work varies according to whether the explanation is formal or material. In the first case, the various examples must be diversified to be able to induce the common mould in which all the gathered observations fit. The hope is that in trying to develop the best mould from the empirical findings we will improve our understanding of the cases being studied. This point of view is taken notably by the social system theory, but it is also shared to a large extent by the social network theory. Most of the observation techniques are qualitative, but we have also seen that statistical patterns can help clarify the configurations of systemic interrelationships. Material theories try to understand phenomena based on a detailed description of the processes from which they stem. This cannot be equated with crude empiricism. To understand sexual behaviour, the description requires conceptual frameworks that point the researcher toward what is most relevant, whether these are the signs that enable one to grasp the meanings that the partners give to their relationship (Ludwig), the phases of the relationship (Bastard, *et al.*), the chain of communication sequences and the place of condom-related behaviour therein (Bastard, *et al.*), bargaining processes (Ferrand and Snijders), etc. This work basically involves informal observation techniques such as semi-structured interviews, etc. It may be systematized through typology work: the development of typologies of problematic situations or behaviour sequences, the revelation of sexual scripts, etc. The feedback from this systematization will then help to construct a theoretical and methodological framework for the next round of research.

Despite the diversity of theoretical perspectives that have been presented in these texts, some general patterns do emerge, namely:

- giving priority to qualitative methods to allow for the singularity of each case and to be able to embrace the cases fully;

- giving the very clear but problematic (see below) predominance of the semi-structured interview;
- showing the concern to reveal the dynamic or process-like natures of phenomena, notably by stressing the narrative aspect of the interviews (the respondent recounts his or her experiences).

On the other hand, the authors are rather vague about the techniques used to analyse the interviews. It seems that, as a rule, the analyses involve a spiral approach in which observations and interpretations follow each other, even interlock, in a process of gradual correction and deepening.

The methods that have been chosen seem to leave the investigators dissatisfied with regard to one essential point, namely, how to discover the interactions from individual interviews. Are the methods up to their theoretical ambitions? Various perspectives have been envisioned, but do not yet seem to have been put into effect, undoubtedly because they raise more problems than they solve. This is especially true of interviewing both partners separately or together, group analyses, and participatory observation in suitable venues, such as bars and saunas. We shall doubtless have to be eclectic here, too, and learn to combine several techniques in order to overcome each technique's limitations. This will call for considerable creativity on the part of researchers in the future. However, we must not be too hasty in putting down individual interviews, which, if they are included in a well-designed study, can provide invaluable, original information. The meagreness of some investigations' findings results more often from a weakness in the way the problem has been stated than from inappropriate investigating techniques.

We have learnt from all this that the search for new theoretical perspectives does not hinge only on the theories' contents. It also involves rethinking the theories' positions within a comprehensive scheme for elucidating reality.

Reference

BERTHELOT, J.-M. (1990) *L'intelligence du social*, Paris: PUF.

Section IV

From Theory to Prevention

Introduction

The three chapters in this last section of the book consider how to incorporate interaction-oriented perspectives into HIV/AIDS prevention programs. Although many previous chapters have emphasized the advantages of interaction-oriented perspectives when trying to influence partners to engage in safer sexual behaviour, this section is different because its focal point is prevention rather than theory. Throughout the book the authors have spoken in many different voices, but three themes emerge: 1) relationships are dynamic processes; 2) the meanings of knowledge, attitudes, beliefs and behaviours are more important than the face-value of each factor in explaining sexual behaviour; 3) behaviours are best understood from the priorities of those engaging in sexual behaviour in contrast to a predefined priority of long life.

In elaborating these themes the authors in this book seem to converge on a similar conclusion. Most recommend that the focus for prevention move away from determining risk groups and attitudes and beliefs related to safer sex, and move toward defining risk situations and the basic values in those situations that reinforce safer sex. Researchers can help those implementing prevention by deconstructing interpersonal situations until the basic values that motivate partners to engage in sexual behaviour are revealed. For example, some basic values discussed in this book are love, pleasure, approval, jealousy, trust and survival. For many partners the same act might be related to different values, while different behaviours may reinforce the same values; condom use may mean mistrust or infidelity to some, and care and love to others. Unprotected sex may mean irresponsibility within one relationship, while it represents commitment and love in another. A negative HIV-test result may mean it is all right to continue past unsafe behaviour to some, while it may mean a warning to start protected sex to others. The key to prevention is understanding when and in what situation the meaning of an action or cognition promotes safer sex and when they inhibit safer sex.

In the first chapter in this section, the Place of Time in Understanding Sexual Behaviour and Designing HIV/AIDS Prevention Programmes, Cohen and Hubert use the concept of *time* to discuss the importance of situational elements. Whether at a societal, individual or interpersonal level they find that time is an omnipresent, if little discussed, component of prevention programs. Several authors in this book have also commented on the dynamic nature of relationships, interaction, and romantic systems. Ferrand and Snijders (Chapter 1) note the dynamic nature of sexuality and that behaviour is, in part, an anticipation of the partner's reaction. That anticipation is based on network norms, prior experiences and some level of verbal or non-verbal bargaining with the partner. Alhemeyer and Ludwig (Chapter 2), and Ingham and van Zessen (Chapter 5) emphasize the temporal nature of communication that is at the heart of intimate systems. Alhemeyer notes that intimate systems are always redefining themselves and adjusting appropriate sexual behaviour in an attempt to maintain themselves. Ingham and van Zessen write that the interaction is the event that triggers other parameters of salience. Bastard, *et al.* (Chapter 3) note nothing is static and suggest that understanding the rules of the game is not sufficient for designing prevention programs, but it is necessary to know when to intervene with an appropriate strategy. Notably, when Bastard, *et al.*, treated their key constructs of fusion-associative and instrumental-reflective as independent variables to predict safer sex, their hypotheses were not confirmed. They explained that the problem probably lay, not in the constructs themselves, but in treating these factors as independent variables in a linear relationship with safer sex. For prevention, these constructs may be more usefully seen as typologies within a sexual situation. The remaining task is to dissect a fusion or associative relationship to find how they affect key values which are related to safer sex.

Like Bastard, *et al.*, several authors in the texts have challenged the direction of the relationship between sexual behaviour and knowledge, attitudes and beliefs. Each author in this section echoes Moatti, *et al.*'s observation that health beliefs can be the cause or the consequence of sexual behaviour. Van Campenhoudt adds that prevention can't assume a hierarchical explanation and that sexual behaviour is interrelated to attitudes, beliefs, cognition and behaviours. For prevention this means that programs will work better if they are designed to reinforce positive behaviour and build community norms for safer sex, rather than build a prevention program with a base of knowledge, attitude and beliefs on the premise that it will yield safer sex behaviour.

In Chapter 12, 'Norms of relationship and normative tensions', Guizzardi recalls the idea of scripts already mentioned several times in the book, particularly in Deven and Meredith (Chapter 9). Scripts serve as a metaphor for sexual behaviour that highlights the importance of situations, timing and partners in developing a prevention program. The concept of scripting sexual behaviour in relationships suggests that sexual behaviour is learned, follows some predefined course over time and has more-or-less room for improvisation. Some scripts are highly structured, actors take their instruction from the director, and parts are well rehearsed. There is no variability over time. Once safer sex is performed there is nothing new to learn, each play is like the one before. Many prevention programs assume relationships follow this types of scripted course. It is assumed that if relationships can be given the proper direction, then safer sex will be the outcome of each interaction. For some limited number of relationships this is true. Once safer sex is learned and rehearsed, it is fixed forever. But for most, at-risk behaviour takes place where the sets, actors, and direction are constantly changing, and those in the least defined relationships have the most room for flexible responses to cues, and much action is ad-lib. The role of the director is not to perfect delivery of preset lines, but to help the actors respond to different situations. Good direction for safer sex scripts is to train the actors to draw on their experience, the particular action on stage, and the other actors' expected response. Life provides the scripts, and prevention programs provide the logistics and direction for the scripts. There are several different types of scripts, from torrid romances to the non-eventful scenes from a long-term marriage; from coming of age sexual adventures to mid-life crisis. Prevention programs must find the appropriate moment when providing the opportunity for safer sex will result in adoption of the recommended behaviour. Once adopted, actors have to rehearse the script until the outcome becomes second nature because they internalize the logic of the script. Consequently, when confronted with a variation in scene or partner, they will know how to adopt the lines to conclude with safer sex. While poor scripts are one reason for failed productions, many more scripts have failed to yield to safer sex because the resources were inadequate (no condoms, lubricant, prevention material, etc.) or there was a poor location, actors were not trained in the appropriate skills, and performances were poorly rehearsed.

Guizzardi, in Chapter 12, focuses on the issue of norms. Most of the other authors' definitions that suggest that a criterion for norms is the acceptance by an individual of a code of behaviour established by a social network or society. Ferrand and Snijders make the distinction between real and perceived norms when they suggest that there are some public values such as fidelity, but the norm, depending on the social network, may be multiple partners. Alhemeyer's definition of norm suggests a kind of internalization. He says that norms are expectations that people are unwilling to learn (in contrast to knowledge), and that when challenged, individuals are forced to make an explanation in the form of apologies or lies. Regardless of the definition of norms, all of the authors agree that their power is derived from the ability to a society, social networks, a partner, or significant others to provide rewards or sanctions. These may be internal and self-regulating such as psychological pleasure, satisfaction, remorse, or guilt or they may be external such as complements or criticism, friendship or loss of friendship, securing a relationships or dissolving a relationship, physical pleasure or pain. In the instance of external sanction, the power of one person or group is a relevant factor.

From a prevention perspective the focus on norms means that intervention must be directed at the relationship, community or the larger society as well as the individual. However, Guizzardi insists on the tensions between the different levels of norms production. Norms are indeed produced by various agents, such as the media, scientists, churches, and politicians, each of whom try to legitimate their perspectives. Guizzardi attempts first of all to elucidate the implicit value system that substends prevention policies and show how it is legitimated. In his opinion, this value system is characterized primarily by technical normativity revolving around condom use and legitimated by medical science. However, Guizzardi ascertains that although these technical norms for prevention appear to be tolerant and rational, they are usually not heeded, which prompts him to wonder to what extent sexual behaviour can be modified through normativization. In answer to this broader question he shows, through references to other texts in this volume, that what is involved is actually a complex system of tensions between various partially autonomous levels (macrosocial processes and institutions, the social network and interpersonal relations, and the individual) that are themselves criss-crossed by tensions that are not necessarily easy to resolve. With regard to institutions in particular Guizzardi stresses the need to study further the role and normative influence of the media. Finally, he observes that the theory of research into sexuality and emotions is plagued by a major problem, namely, that the research approaches continue to be highly rational. Chapters 5, 6 and 7 have drawn attention to this aspect of individual-centred approaches. However, Guizzardi claims that a rational vision of the problems at hand continues to permeate the relational and social context-oriented approaches that are proposed in this volume.

The last chapter, 'New conceptual perspectives and prevention', by Hausser summarizes the preceding chapters. He observes that the AIDS epidemic and promoting less risky behaviour are complex social phenomena that defy easy solutions. Hausser makes a significant contribution to the book by categorizing the ideological frameworks behind many current prevention models and suggests that they create blinkers that often limit the public response to HIV/AIDS. Expanding on Guizzardi's text, he finds that the most common model of HIV prevention is the biomedical model that promotes the value of long life above everything else. Longevity is promoted, in a free market economy, by assuming that individuals, when informed of the risk and ways to prevent danger, will make a rational choice for longer life. While this free market ideology does not absolve the government from responsibility, it suggests that the role of governments is to provide information that enables the consumer to remain healthy. The responsibility of the public is to make the right choice. Hausser notes that this overlooks quality of life decisions that individuals and partners make regarding their lives and sexuality. For many, improved quality of life may not include safer sex, and as Cohen and Hubert indicate in the first chapter of this section, safer sex may be very low on the list of priorities of sexual partners.

Hausser suggests several different implications for prevention at the end of his chapter. To expand on one point, the current emphasis on the individual ignores the role of many structural elements, such as poverty, sexism, education, hunger, poor access to resources, war and immigration. Cohen and Hubert note how these current social trends can have a large impact on the spread of HIV. The question is what proportion of the prevention resources should be diverted to solve more intrinsic social inequities that have an impact on the epidemic and what level of resources should be spent on specific HIV/AIDS prevention programs.

This section does not proscribe a set prevention program under the interaction-oriented perspective. Rather it warns that prevention programs, like the epidemic, need to evolve, consider relationships, and veer away from direct advocacy of non-risky behaviour, be it condoms, fidelity, abstinence, or mutual testing. The theoretical findings and prevention advice offered in this book run parallel courses. Researchers would understand sexual behaviour better if they understood the meaning behind the action, the interactional processes and the social contexts in which they take place. Similarly, prevention could be improved if preventers listened to the priorities of the populations at risk, developed programs that met their needs, and understood that prevention has to coordinate societal, community, individual, and partner interventions.

Chapter 11

The Place of Time in Understanding Sexual Behaviour and Designing HIV/ AIDS Prevention Programs

Mitchell Cohen and Michel Hubert

Introduction

Many communities[1] throughout the world are battling an AIDS epidemic where sexual intercourse is a major mode of transmission. Until a vaccine is developed, one goal of HIV/AIDS prevention programs is to reduce the future impact of AIDS by influencing present sexual behaviour. Identifying those factors related to the adoption and maintenance of safer sex is one goal of HIV/AIDS prevention research. Once identified, HIV/AIDS prevention programs can develop interventions with individuals, partners and communities that emphasize those factors related to behaviour change. The purposes of this chapter are to demonstrate that time is a crucial concept in understanding sexual behaviour, and to suggest ways that increase the effectiveness of interventions by considering the place of time.

Table 11.1 Perspective of time and sexual behaviour

Level	Time perspective
Society and community	Intergeneration transmission of cultural norms
	Intrageneration current trends and life-styles
	Stages of the HIV epidemic
Individual	Rational assessment of health outcome
	Sequence of developmental stages
	Life cycle phases
Partnership interactions	Sequence of interactions between peers and partners

Sexual intercourse occurs between partners at a particular moment in time. While one explanation of why partners engage in unsafe sexual intercourse[2] is *the heat of the moment,* understanding sexual behaviour requires investigating more than that instant in time when partners engage in sex. The type and frequency of sex depend upon societal pressures, individual needs and processes, and partner interactions that precede a particular sexual act. Table 11.1 displays different perspectives of time for each of these levels.

Time: Society and Community

Intergenerational Transmission of Cultural Norms

Time, in the context of sexual cultural norms, represents an intergenerational consistency of sexual patterns and behaviour. When designing an HIV/AIDS prevention program directed at modifying sexual behaviour, authorities are frequently advised to 'be culturally sensitive'. This is shorthand for the recognition that traditions, customs and sexual norms are key factors in understanding patterns of sexual intercourse.

Images of sexuality and sexual behaviour vary, not only from one society to the next, but also between generations with a given society. (see Deven and Meredith, Chapter 8 for a more in-depth discussion of culture). In many communities the traditional practices of sex often conflict with the AIDS prevention advice to use condoms or to engage in non-penetrative sex or to stay faithful to a lifetime single partner. For example, having many children and/or having multiple partners is often associated with positive attributes such as potency, power, vigor and fertility. In turn these attributes translate into increased status within social networks. Even for those who are HIV-positive, the value of raising children is often much higher than the threat of perinatal infection or the perception of infertility. In many communities in Africa an infertile woman often faces isolation from the community, the loss of a husband or the inability to attract a spouse (Hardy, 1988; Lallement, *et al.*, 1992). Also, depending on the social norms, social networks and individual desires, the value of fidelity is often outweighed by the pleasure and status conveyed by multiple partners. Given the central importance of child bearing and the social status associated with fertility, communities with strong values of procreation and/or multiple sexual partners are likely to be less responsive to most AIDS prevention messages.

Traditional sexual norms do change over time. As societies become more mobile, urbanized children are more likely to be an economic and social burden than an asset. Among urban dwellers, there is evidence of a desire for smaller families and a greater emphasis on sex for pleasure without procreation. The moral debate surrounding AIDS prevention recommendations on safer sex is part of the continuing social debate about the acceptability of sex for pleasure and the role of fidelity. This debate is witnessed in many forums such as the church, the media, music videos, advertising, and government. Where the popular media, music and advertising use sexual images as a lure for the purchase of products, it is likely to be a subcontext that sex for pleasure is a widely accepted norm. Without judging the merits of the moralists' point of view, from an empirical viewpoint, individuals in communities that have a norm of sexual intercourse for pleasure rather than procreation are more likely to adopt safer sex because there is less conflict in normative values. (See Ahlemeyer and Ludwig, Chapter 2, for additional reasons why sex-for-pleasure hedonistic systems or prostitutive systems are more likely to adopt safer sex.)

The impact of cultural norms on the spread of HIV has been documented in several societies. For example, in some central African societies men traditionally prefer women having a dry vagina during intercourse. This leaves women more susceptible to lacerations that facilitate transmission of HIV (Ankra, 1990; Hardy, 1988). Another example is that in some tribes in Western Africa, there is a time-honored tradition where the brother-in-law adopts the wife of a deceased brother and consummates the adoption with sexual intercourse. This practice is particularly likely to increase the spread of HIV because many husbands' deaths are now due to AIDS. A third example found in many cultures ranging from the urban centers of the US and Norway, the villages of Rwanda, and the islands of the South Pacific is the association of semen exchange with intimacy, power, and love (Herdt, 1982; Prieur, 1990). This value greatly limits the use of condoms, even with high awareness that they reduce the risk of AIDS (Taylor, 1990).

Religion is among the most powerful channels of intergenerational transmission of values, and some social networks object to the use of condoms because their religion prohibits the use of contraceptives. In one instance, in Tanzania, the understanding of this cultural constraint led to a redefinition of condom use. Muslim clergy redefined it from contraception to a method of disease prevention. In that context the religious leaders could encourage their followers to use condoms. For orthodox Catholics the Pope's directive against artificial methods of contraception and his advocacy of procreation creates a conflict between disease prevention and loyalty to the church. For those with strong religious beliefs and support structures, this creates a significant barrier to adopting condoms.

Different cultural values related to homosexuality can greatly affect the effectiveness of HIV prevention programs. While self-defined gay communities are a fairly recent phenomenon of the twentieth century, homosexual behaviour has a long tradition. For example, on the Kalepo Island, New Guinea, homosexual behaviour is part of a rite of passage where younger men are initiated with the semen of older men (Gray, 1985). In Latin and South America, homosexuality is practised in a larger sexual repertoire that includes bisexuality and frequently the insertive partner is not viewed as gay. This *machismo* behaviour coexists with exclusively homosexual and transvestite subcultures (Parker and Tawil, 1991). When groups migrate from one country to another country, many sexual customs continue. The finding by Carrier Magana and Raul (1991) and Parker and Tawil (1991) that the homosexuality of African- and Mexican-American men differs considerably from that of Anglo-American men is consistent with other studies of ethnic populations that have shown differences in sexual behaviour between ethnic populations within the same country.

An obstacle to HIV/AIDS prevention is the historical moralist position against homosexuality. As shown in Figure 11.1, in Europe there remains a considerable feeling that homosexuality is never justified, particularly in Portugal, Ireland, and Italy. Frequently moralists argue that AIDS is divine punishment for deviant or sinful behaviour. Some prevention programs incorporate their views but argue that even if the punishment is just, permitting AIDS to spread will affect innocent victims, and therefore has to be controlled. Countering this argument, human rights advocates believe that the right to health services is universal and includes HIV prevention and care. The notion that there is divine attribution is unacceptable. Everyone at risk is morally equivalent – there are no innocent victims.

Another example of a cultural bias that serves as a barrier to HIV/AIDS prevention is the belief by many health educators that only homosexuals engage in anal intercourse. Yet anal intercourse is practised between heterosexuals in many communities, where it functions as a form of birth control, sexual pleasure and rite of passage (Agrafiotis, 1990; Spira, Bajos and le Groupe ACSF, 1993). In Tanzania, according to a health educator at the National AIDS Control Program, some individuals have adopted the practise of anal sex as a way of preventing AIDS because prevention messages have mentioned only unprotected vaginal intercourse as risky sexual behaviour.

The prevention message from the focus on intergenerational norms is that norms can serve as facilitators or inhibitors to HIV/AIDS prevention programs and that there are different agents which actively perpetuate normative values. A general rule is, where possible and ethical, integrate and adapt HIV-prevention programs within existing cultural norms so that they are complementary and recruit the services of the agents of normative values to assist in HIV prevention. This is generally more effective than establishing counter-cultural or entirely new values in a community and creating new channels for the diffusion of new values. There are, however, times when HIV prevention carries a political or social agenda of empowering different at-risk groups, such as women, even in cultures where this is not the norm. For example, empowering women as a prevention strategy is based on the belief that if women participate more equally in sexual decisions and have more power in a relationship the result will be safer sexual behaviour. For

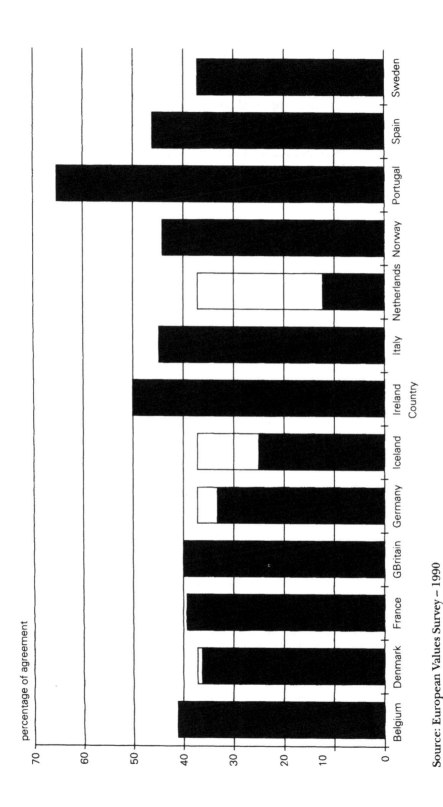

percentage of agreement

Source: European Values Survey – 1990

Figure 11.1 Homosexuality is never justified

both men and women, this strategy involves a complex program of changing norms and sexual behaviours.

Intrageneration Social and Political Trends

Current trends and events are often countervailing forces to long held traditional norms. Every new generation confronts unique technologies, crises and political events. In response new life-styles may be adopted (Attias-Donfut, 1988). Medical technology has been a reason for a change in sexual norms. The invention of the pill and widespread diffusion of antibiotics had a large impact on the generation defining their sexuality in the late 1960s and early 1970s, particularly in developed nations. These medical innovations allowed the valorization of free love with multiple sexual partners, open marriage and other counter-cultural sexual experimentation.

Social policy has an impact on each generaion. For example, starting in the 1960s there was a marked liberalization of policies in North America and western Europe of laws prohibiting gay men from meeting in public places. The subsequent increased sexual networking in saunas and venues for sexual intercourse was seen as evidence of a more open self-proclamation of gay identity. Unfortunately, these venues provided the perfect environment for the spread of HIV. Fortunately, those factors that led to rapid transmission of HIV also led to rapid diffusion of information through defined social and communication networks and this contributed to the success of HIV/AIDS prevention programs in gay communities (Abramson and Herdt, 1990; Connell *et al.*, 1991; Stall and Paul, 1989). In the 1990s one expression of improved civil liberties in eastern Europe is the liberalization of laws forbidding homosexuality. In these communities information about HIV and AIDS has been limited and greater sexual activity has accompanied new-found freedom (Prochazka, 1994). A dramatic increase in HIV infection is highly probable unless major intervention programs are begun. However, as Pollak in France (1991) and Kelly (1990) in the US suggest, there are diverse norms within different gay communities and many men who have sex with other men do not identify with a gay community. For HIV prevention to be effective, an understanding of the social networks and normative values will facilitate creating effective programs.

Political struggles unique to each generation can effect behavior. The drug culture that grew in the 1960s and 1970s and the increase in injecting drug use populations during that period caused a tremendous increase in HIV infection because of the efficient transmission of HIV through shared needles or solutions and the exploitation of sex to earn money or barter for drugs (Fullilove, 1992). The expansion of drug use starting in the 1960s can be traced to the larger international political conflicts. During the cold war drug money was used to finance clandestine political and military opposition in the south-east Mediterranean, south-east and north-east Asia and South America. Drug suppliers found a ready market in both the urban ghettos of developed countries and among the large middle class baby boom generation in their late teens and early twenties. Over the past few decades drug producers and cartels have developed and expanded an industry. Drug use is spreading, as drug entrepreneurs find it easier to cross borders and demand is rising in southern and eastern Europe. Drug suppliers thrive upon the poor and disenfranchised as they offer substantial economic benefits to those engaged in the drug trade, including distributors in low income areas who have few other economic opportunities. While drug treatment and needle exchange programs have proven effective in decreasing the spread of HIV infection (Des Jarlais and Friedman, 1989), programs that provide alternative economic and social opportunities for those economies that are dependent on drugs are likely to be part of a longer term solution to halting the spread of AIDS through injecting drug use.

Wars, famine and poverty are crises faced by each generation that result in a greater risk of HIV infection. Migration patterns where families are uprooted from their traditional support groups often result in changing sexual norms. The increased supply of un- and under-employed urban inhabitants and an expanding network of sex workers in both developed and developing countries result in more venues and opportunities for sex. Epidemics of STDs, including AIDS, often follow military campaigns where there is a lively market for commercial sex workers. Nguma (1992) tells how the border conflict between Tanzania and Uganda produced the key situational factors for the rapid spread of HIV: the available money from the highly mobile soldiers, truck drivers and black market entrepreneurs created a great demand for sexual partners. The active sexual networks, combined with great mobility and the introduction of the virus, led to the rapid and widespread transmission of HIV in eastern Africa.

The instability in eastern Europe is, in many ways, analogous to the experiences of eastern Africa. The disintegration of the Soviet Union, the widespread migration patterns and the numerous armed conflicts throughout eastern Europe and the former Soviet Republics are likely to provide fertile ground for the rapid spread of HIV. Some young women and men migrating to urban centres find that sex work is the only means of survival, and their immediate needs of shelter, food and money far outweigh their perceived threat from AIDS. While commercial sex workers range from willing participants to those who are exploited by sex entrepreneurs, clearly sex workers and their clients who engage in unprotected sex are at high risk of HIV infection.

It would be tragic to allow HIV to become widespread among migrant populations, those displaced during war and within emerging gay communities. After ten years, prevention experts can provide the methods to mount effective prevention programs. Nevertheless, the many higher priorities of governments, lack of experience with community-based organizations (CBOs), and poor economic conditions, are likely to mean the rapid spread of HIV among populations in high risk situations.

Stages of the HIV Epidemic

The relationship between sexual behavior and the AIDS epidemic is two-way. The AIDS epidemic, as reported by the media and experienced by communities, is itself a crisis that has caused changes in traditional sexual behaviour over the past decade. Time, here, is the underlying dimension in the stages of the HIV epidemic. Cohen (1991) describes four stages of the HIV epidemic: the beginning stage of the HIV epidemic when the virus is introduced; the peaking stage when the HIV epidemic has peaked in a particular community; the declining stage, as the incidence of HIV infection declines; and the tail stage where the epidemic continues to infect the community at a relatively low level. The concept of time underlying the stages of the epidemic is not calendar time, but time associated with the progression of the epidemic in a community. In Figure 11.2, the epidemic patterns for the San Francisco and Amsterdam gay cohorts are shown, and the same stage in each community corresponds to different years and lasts for different periods of time. These patterns suggest substantially different behavioural patterns which resulted in a sharp increase and equally sharp decline in HIV incidence in San Francisco while there was as slower increase and slower decline in Amsterdam. Even within the same country, different communities (as represented by neighbourhoods, ethnic identification, sexual orientation, etc.) may have different HIV epidemics.

Cohen and Chwalow (1993) suggest that different factors are related to changing to safer sex during different stages of the epidemic (see Table 11.2), and communities could maximize their prevention efforts by designing programs that emphasize those factors most related to change during a specific stage. The overall message from this analysis is that policy, community and normative factors are among the most important in promoting safer sex throughout the epidemic, and these are briefly discussed in this section. The personality and information processing frameworks are discussed later in this chapter.

Unlike other epidemics where the medical consequences are quickly apparent, communities see few AIDS cases in the beginning stage of the HIV epidemic, due to the time lag between HIV infection and manifestation of AIDS. Newly seropositive individuals place few demands for prevention or health care services on families, partners, their community or governments, and consequently the impact of awareness of PWAs and those who are HIV positive is low. Still, awareness of the pandemic is high, in part due to the international response to AIDS from the World Health Organization and

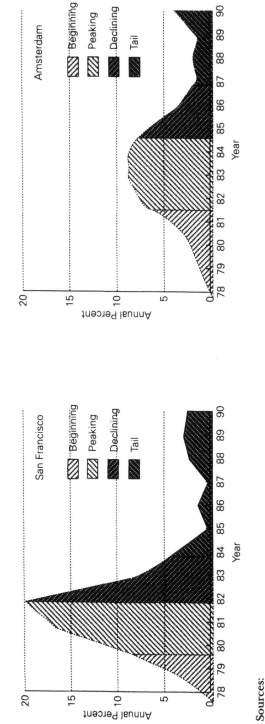

Sources:

Amsterdam: van Griensven (1988), deWit, *et al.* (1991); N=1431; 685 Hepatitis B vaccine trial; recruited between November 1980 and November 1982, and 746 healthy homosexual men recruited October 1984 onwards from homosexual communities.

San Francisco: Hessol, *et al.* (1989) and personal correspondence. N=320; Hepatitis B vaccine trial; recruited through San Francisco City Clinic; seronegative for Hepatitis B at recruitment.

Figure 11.2   Stages of the HIV epidemic: annual HIV infection

Table 11.2 Changing to safer sex: relative contribution of factors over stages of the epidemic

	Stages of the HIV epidemic			
	Beginning	Peaking	Declining	Tail
Personality factors				
Self-efficacy	moderate	moderate-low	moderate-low	low
ID with community	moderate	moderate	moderate	moderate-low
Intimacy (negative relation)	moderate	moderate	high	high
Information processing factors				
Aware of HIV-/PWA	low	high	moderate	low
KAB of safer sex	moderate	moderate	moderate-low	low
Awareness of serostatus	moderate-low	moderate-low	low	low
Normative factors				
Partner/peer interaction	moderate	moderate-high	high	high
Policy and community factors				
Government policy	moderate	high	high	high
Community cohesion	moderate	high	high	high

international non-governmental organizations (NGOs). Most governments acted swiftly to insure the safety of blood supplies, but there is usually a far more moderate response regarding prevention during the beginning stages of the epidemic (Cohen, *et al.*, 1992).

There were many reasons for the slow government response to AIDS. Particularly in developing countries, the lack of response during the initial stage was because other health priorities and more immediate life-threatening diseases drained the resources of the public health agencies. A second reason was the battle for the type of HIV prevention between the *moralists* and the *pragmatists*. The moralists tend to suggest the culpability of certain groups and advocate sexual abstinence, long-term fidelity, and legal punishment for perceived abnormal behaviour. The pragmatists tend to offer risk-reduction techniques such as condom use and nonpenetrative safer sex techniques (Clift and Stears, 1991; Kaplan, 1990; Wellings, 1991). Other reasons include institutionalized homophobia, lack of urgency, bureaucratic battling and difficulty confronting social taboos. Also the slow implementation of policy affecting the rights of HIV-positive individuals to access housing, health care, and insurance were often inadequate to neutralize the discrimination against them (Tomasevski, 1992). As a result many individuals avoided prevention programs that they felt would label them as HIV positive.

In many communities the first individuals to respond to the epidemic were those who had a strong sense of self-efficacy and who adopted safer sex in response to their perceived risk. A few of those individuals had a strong affiliation with their community and started community-based organizations (CBOs) and AIDS service organizations (ASOs). These organizations tended to fill gaps left by the inadequate response by governments. During the initial period of the epidemic, the most effective response came from those CBOs which perceived a threat to their constituencies and designed programs to emphasize empowerment and self-efficacy. Over the stages of the epidemic, the strategies of community organizations were likely to shift from reinforcing self-efficacy to providing networks for peers and applying social pressure for change. As these organizations grew, they encouraged a greater sense of community identification and contributed to peer networks where safer sex became the norm (Kippax, *et al.*, 1990). Often these initial ASOs evolved into major HIV prevention and care organizations (Cohen, 1992; O'Malley, 1992). Governments funded them to provide HIV/AIDS prevention in recognition of their expertise and rapport within communities at risk and as a way of distancing themselves from directly recommending risk reduction methods such as condoms or clean needles.

Over the period of the epidemic, public information campaigns developed by governments and CBOs helped to inform the population about AIDS; most surveys indicate that the mass media was a primary source of information about AIDS for the general population. Evidence from hotlines throughout the developed countries indicates that major news stories and major HIV/AIDS-prevention campaigns spark public concern and response. For example, the death of movie star Rock Hudson from AIDS, the HIV infection of sports superstar Magic Johnson, or the tainted blood supply in France placed AIDS on the public agenda (Brown, 1992). While increasing public awareness is often the goal of public HIV/AIDS prevention programs, the coverage by the mass media is not always positive or in the best interest of public health. If the past is a guide, the media will rarely cover AIDS consistently during the initial stages of the epidemic, and then only from a predominantly moral and medical perspective (Albert, 1988; Herzlich and Pierret, 1989). For example the stereotyping by the media of injecting drug users and gays as those mostly affected by HIV provided a convenient rationalization for the general population – 'I'm not one of those' – and led to their continued high risk sexual behaviour. To the extent that HIV/AIDS is perceived as a serious, real and immediate threat by individuals and communities, sexual behaviour change is likely to be adopted. To the degree that safer sex is perceived as 'the other community's problem' or a vehicle by one part of the community to suppress another part the result is likely to be the continuation of long held sexual norms which provide a continued fertile ground for the spread of HIV. For example, viewing safer sex advice as a form of genocide by some African communities or as contraction of personal freedom by some gay communities led to denial by some community members that AIDS was a real threat.

In general, effective HIV-prevention recommendations have largely been the domain of advertisements, brochures, billboards and other promotional, rather than editorial, aspects of the media. Even here unrealistic alarms may be counterproductive. For example, the highly awarded Grim Reaper campaign in Australia caused an overwhelming response by the public to get tested, but the risk portrayed to the general public far exceeded the actual danger of the epidemic and thus lost credibility and may, in the end, stifle change towards safer sex among specific communities at risk (Dwyer, *et al.*, 1988). Another instance of poor practices following effective information dissemination is found in many communities in Africa where mature men seek intercourse with very young women because they fear contracting AIDS from older partners. Because many of the men are already infected, the undesired result is a rising epidemic among very young women, but there is little doubt that the motivation for this new behaviour was a desire by men to avoid infection.

Few western communities have entered the tail stage of the epidemic. Among the gay communities that have entered this stage, the maintenance of safer sex has been difficult (Stall, *et al.*, 1992). Typically there has been reduced funding for the affected community during this stage even as evidence of increasing infection rates mounts. In general, during the declining stage of the epidemic, HIV-prevention programs have attempted to influence the more difficult to reach populations who are less involved with community-based organization. Consequently, ASOs have expanded their roles or governments have started programs targeted towards underserved individuals.

Individual and partner interaction factors such as information processing, need for intimacy and partner negotiation also play a dynamic role over the stages of the epidemic. These are discussed below.

Time: The Individual

Rational Assessment of Outcomes

Central to several theories of sexual behaviour is the idea that individuals, over time, try to optimize their outcomes. From this cognitive perspective, sexual behaviour is the result of an assessment of the risk of AIDS and some combination of knowledge, attitudes and beliefs. A frequently cited optimization theory in AIDS prevention research is the Health Belief Model (HBM); there has been considerable research directed towards the goal of proving or disproving it (Moatti and Pollak, 1990; Moatti, *et al.*, Chapter 6; Robert and Rosser, 1990). Like other cost-benefit models, the HBM suggests that individuals will optimize their long-term outcome by making a rational choice to adopt safer sex once they understand that:

- they are susceptible to the HIV infection;
- HIV infection leads to the fatal disease AIDS;
- through safer sex HIV can be avoided;
- they have the resources to adopt safer sex.

Notably, for these theories to be relevant, sexual behaviour must be under the control of the individual, and populations at risk for HIV often do not meet that condition.

From the perspective of time, HIV-prevention programs that use cognitive models have often failed because they assume that AIDS prevention is a central priority. Yet many people have more immediate needs that take precedence over long-term and uncertain outcomes of unprotected sex. Love and intimacy, partner and peer approval, and economic need are powerful pressures towards unsafe sex. For example, an individual might ask him- or herself what is more important: My health in ten years or falling in love tonight? Using a condom to protect my health or not raising suspicions about infidelity? The chance of getting AIDS or feeding my family? The chance of getting AIDS or being made fun of by my peers?

Even if the HBM were to work as suggested by their authors, and the possibility of contracting HIV and AIDS motivated persons to change, it has proven extremely difficult for individuals to correctly perceive their susceptibility and the severity of the AIDS and/or admit that the long-term consequence of infection leads to a fatal disease (Montgomery, *et al.*, 1989; Weinstein, 1989).

On a more methodological level, Moatti and Pollak (1990) criticize the sequence of cause and effect hypothesized by the Health Belief Model. They suggest that knowledge, attitudes and beliefs are as much a consequence of behaviour as the cause of behaviour; they note that correlation analysis used to prove the theory may actually represent rationalizations for behaviour. In short, they say that the HBM has confused the time sequence of what comes first, the behaviour or the attitudes.

Bandura's (1988) social cognitive theory (SCT) differs from the HBM by adding the component of self-efficacy. It suggests that the individual's perceived ability that he or she can successfully execute safer sexual practices is a major factor in adopting safer sex. While SCT allows for a person to be motivated to change his or her sexual behaviour because of the realization of long-term consequences of risk behaviour, in the short-term SCT recognizes that peers and partners play an important role because they allow an individual to learn through observation and modeling. Consequently, sexual behaviour change can be explained as a short-term imitation of behaviour as well as a more distant calculated way to avoid AIDS. Evidence from San Francisco (Frutchey, 1989) and other communities (Boer, *et al.*, 1991, de Vries, Dijkstra and Kuhlman, 1988) demonstrates that group discussions and workshops increase self-efficacy through skills enhancement and provide social support and modeling from peers. Both are important in promoting change.

While optimization models have been legitimately criticized, HIV/AIDS programs based on disseminating information and changing attitudes can be successful if they are introduced at the appropriate time in the epidemic. During the initial and peaking stages of the HIV epidemic, information heightens anxiety. Not everyone responds to anxiety in the same fashion. Many reduce their anxiety by adopting safer sex or seeking information which may then lead to safer sex. Others reduce anxiety by cognitive defense mechanisms such as rationalizing their behaviour as not risky ('I only have sex with people I know') or tuning out undesired messages. Still others may welcome participation in a risky situation. Finally, some may become fatalistic and continue with unsafe sex with full knowledge of the risk. (Guizzardi, in Chapter 12, elaborates on these mechanisms in his typology of responses to the risk of AIDS.) In most relatively tight social and sexual networks, basic information about unsafe sex seems to reach a saturation level by the peaking stage. However, during the declining and tail stages unsafe sex is related to negative attitudes about condoms and misperceptions about the efficacy of different preventive methods (Cohen and Chwalow, 1993). For example, there continue to be considerable misperceptions about infection through casual contact and the efficacy of short-term monogamy. If a person feels that he or she can contract AIDS through casual contact, then why stop unprotected sexual intercourse? If a person feels he or she is practising safer sex by maintaining a short-term monogamous relationship, then why adopt other measures?

Not all information is created equal, and certain types of information are likely to motivate behaviour change more than others. For example, a prevention strategy undertaken by many communities is to advocate the knowledge of serostatus through HIV testing and counseling. The belief is that those who find they are HIV positive will stop having unsafe sex and those who find they are negative will start having safer sex. Although there is considerable evidence that, early in the epidemic, knowledge of serostatus, particularly combined with counseling, can increase the rate of change to safer sex, it seems to make little difference in adopting safer sex at the tail of the epidemic (Casadonte, *et al.*, 1990; Connell, *et al.*, 1989; Frazer, *et al.*, 1988; Huggins, *et al.*, 1991). There has been little research done on using testing as a means to promote safer sex among stable partners. Potentially, testing could be one strategy to promote safer behaviour among mutually monogamous partners. Regardless of the impact of knowledge of serostatus on prevention, an anonymous testing program may be useful to identify HIV-positive persons and give them an option for early treatment.

Many working in AIDS prevention feel that the main motivator for sexual behaviour change will be personal awareness of someone infected with HIV or dying of AIDS. Studies indicate that, in communities that have reached the peaking stage, awareness of a friend or partner with AIDS or who is HIV positive is likely to have a relatively larger impact on behaviour change as it underlines personal vulnerability to HIV infection (Cohen and Chwalow, 1993). However, it is clearly false that the change to safer sex is simply a function of people becoming aware of persons with AIDS or seropositive status. There is ample evidence showing that many persons who are aware of persons with AIDS (PWAs) and HIV-positive persons continue unsafe practices. While some of these unprotected practices may be a conscious decision among partners of the same HIV status, the recent increase in HIV incidence within gay communities in several western urban centers indicates that simply knowing someone is insufficient motivation for maintaining safer sex.

In general, the trend over the epidemic reflects a diminishing impact of information and individual decision-making and a heightening impact of strategies that use peer, partner and community pressure towards safer sex. Prevention programs have been more effective when they evolve from providing information to an emphasis on group prevention sessions, safer-sex workshops, participation in programs and other forms of interactive strategies.

Sequence of Developmental Stages

Most cognitive models place their emphasis on some assessment of outcomes by an individual. In the area of HIV/AIDS research the distant negative outcome of AIDS is what motivates persons to change their behaviour. Static cognitive theories suggest similar outcomes given the same knowledge, attitudes and beliefs. In contrast, developmental theories focus on sequential changes in the psychological structure of the individual which would cause him or her to interpret information differently.

Catania, Kegeles and Coates's (1990) AIDS Risk Reduction Model (ARRM) introduces the importance of stages of decision-making in adopting safer sex. The ARRM starts with the same criteria as most other cognitive models. Individuals perceive the risk of HIV infection based on their sexual behaviour. From that point it diverges from static models by emphasizing three stages of decision-making rather than estimating static levels of knowledge, attitudes and beliefs. The three stages are labeling high-risk behaviour as problematic, making a commitment to changing high-risk behaviour, and engaging in safer sex. The three stages are shown in Table 11.3.

Catania does not speculate on the variation in the time it takes individuals to move through the stages, nor does he believe these stages are universal. However, he does suggest that HIV-prevention programs can facilitate the passage from one stage to the next by introducing moderate levels of anxiety,

Table 11.3 Stages of the AARM model

Stages	Hypothesized influences	Outcome indicators
Labeling	Susceptibility; transmission knowledge; aversion emotions; social factors	Risk assessment for becoming HIV +
Commitment	Aversive emotions; perceptions of enjoyment; risk reduction; self-efficacy; social factors	Intention to engage in safer sex in 'x' weeks
Enactment	Aversive emotions; sexual communications; help-seeking; social factors	Practicing safer sex

developing external motivation such as public health programs, and encouraging social networks to provide support for safer sex.

Life Cycle Phases

Peto, *et al.* (1992) suggest that individuals pass through life cycle phases. Each phase implies specific roles and expectations, imposes specific responsibilities and determines specific opportunities and constraints that may have an impact on sexual behaviours and attitudes towards HIV risk. The phases include

- discovery of sexuality and love;
- the search for a way of life and partner;
- stabilization of a relationship;
- deterioration of a relationship; and
- the life of a person who lives without a primary relationship.

The phases refer to the individuals' emotional, sexual and/or marital history. They focus on social attributes over time rather than on information processing and optimization of outcomes suggested by most cognitive models. While every individual starts with the first phase, the remaining four do not necessarily follow a determined sequence. These phases are further discussed in Bastard, *et al.*, Chapter 3.

The existence of life cycle stages has received some empirical support in the domains of personal growth (Sheehy, 1976) and religion (Kohlberg, 1983), and is being tested in the realm of HIV/AIDS (Hubert, *et al.*, 1993; Laumann, *et al.*, 1994). Hypothetically, during the discovery phase, knowledge and self-efficacy to engage in safer sex are likely to be low. Individuals who have intercourse during this early phase have a drive to explore sex and often there is a cultural expectation to find love. Both place individuals at risk because they are more vulnerable to their partners' wishes and less interested in the probability of contracting AIDS. For them, HIV infection is an additional concern in an already difficult period of maturation.

As the individual enters the second phase of searching for a way of life and partner, many continue to be at risk. As stable relations become a possibility for an individual, suggesting the use of a condom may be seen as a sign of lack of trust, an indication of infidelity, or an obstacle to love. Ideally, if the environment were supportive, safer sex would be part of the negotiation about becoming sexually involved. Unfortunately this is rarely the case, and the desire to search for a partner may require unsafe sex as a statement of trust and love.

During the stable relationship phase the number of partners is limited and there is less sexual experimentation. Consequently, the individual is at low risk of becoming HIV positive. Some risk continues. While a person may be monogamous, past behaviour may have infected one partner, and unprotected sex often occurs before the serostatus of the partners is known. Also, it is not uncommon for at least one partner to have sexual relations outside their primary relationship (Hubert, *et al.*, 1993; Johnson, *et al.*, 1992; Johnson, *et al.*, 1994; Spira, *et al.*, 1993; van Zessen, and Sandfort, 1991). In cultures allowing multiple marriages or which place a value on multiple partners, this phase may continue to have substantial risk of contracting HIV.

As relationships dissolve and one or both partners re-enter the sexual marketplace, there is again a heightened risk. There is some indication (Hubert, *et al.*, 1993) that although most of these partners are knowledgeable about HIV and AIDS, the habits of unprotected sex practiced in a stable relationship are difficult to break and the lack of familiarity with condoms and other types of safer sex leave those reentering the sexual market more likely to have unsafe sex.

The idea of individuals going through defined temporal phases opens avenues for new research. If prevention programs can identify the situations surrounding each phase, then messages targeted towards modifying risky behaviour typical of each phase can be developed.

Time: Peer and Partner Interaction

Several theories suggest behaviour is the result of an interaction between peers and partners. Virtually every study that has measured the impact of partner and peer interaction has found it significantly related to sexual behaviour (Hunt and Davies, 1991; Kelly, *et al.*, 1989; Valdiserri, 1991; Weisman, *et al.*, 1989). Several theories suggest the reasons why partners and peers have such a strong influence. Each, however, requires a sequence of interactions and an expectation of an outcome. In addition, the stage of the relationship is a significant factor in understanding the type of sexual behaviour.

Unlike the long-term negative outcome of contracting AIDS, interactions often result in immediate incentives for safer or unsafe sex. Social acceptance and the gratification of pleasing others, or the equally immediate negative outcomes of social rejection and isolation are powerful motivators (see Ferrand and Snijders, Chapter 1). The immediate reward of social acceptance underpins many behaviour modification programs, where peer pressure and public commitment are used to change strong habitual (or addictive) behaviour, and peer support is used to reinforce change (Hergenhahn, 1982).

Partners and peers can also be role models. After personal experience, the most powerful stimuli often come from social groups, peers and sexual partners, rather than stemming from personal awareness of information (Bandura, 1977b; Guizzardi, *et al.*, Chapter 9; Rosenstock, Strecher and Becker, 1988). Theories, such as Heider's (1958) balance theory, predict that behaviour will continue unaltered until it is challenged, for example by a disagreement between peers or partners. There is clear evidence that the best predictor of unsafe sex is the previous practice of unsafe sex (Connell, *et al.*, 1989; Martin, 1986; McCusker, *et al.*, 1989a). From Heider's perspective this would be an understood behaviour between two partners, and, unless there was a disagreement causing imbalance, the *status quo* behaviour would be likely to continue. Once there was disagreement, the partner with the greatest influence would be likely to persuade or coerce the other into safe or unsafe sex.

Attribution theory (Heider, 1958; Memon, 1991) and Social Interaction Theory (Friedman, Levine and Siegel, 1986; McGuire, 1991) suggests that behaviour can be explained in terms of one partner's perception or expectation of the other regarding safe or unsafe sex. For example, if one partner believes the other would interpret condom use as admitting to infidelity, condoms would not be used even if in reality he or she would welcome the suggestion (Peto, *et al.*, 1992). The power of partners is suggested from many studies that show that more unsafe sex occurs within a primary relationship than between partners who are not in a primary relationship or between individuals who also have sex outside their primary relationship (Bye, 1987; Connell, *et al.*, 1988; McCusker, *et al.*, 1989b; Martin, *et al.*, 1989). In relationships, this perspective suggests the importance of clarifying expectations with a partner and, in some instances, negotiating safer sex before unsafe practices become the default behaviour.

Another interpersonal interpretation of sexual behaviour hypothesizes that different sexual behaviours are related to stages of a relationship. Peto, *et al.* (1992) suggests three stages: seduction; familiarity; ending. During seduction the more passionate the relationship is, the less probable the use of condoms. During the stage of familiarity the partners are more secure in their relationship and feel safer, and the use of condoms is less likely even if they had been used at the beginning of the relationship. Within the first months of a relationship the level of security that is necessary to engage in unprotected sex is often reached (Frank, 1992; Lenneer-Axelson, 1988). During the end of a relationship, partners are unlikely to use condoms if they have not been part of their sexual practice in the past. During this stage there is a greater likelihood of multiple partners.

Discussion and Conclusions

Before AIDS, *safer* or *unsafe* sex carried little meaning. Today, *safer sex* translates into one of the few ways to decrease the rate of HIV infection. HIV/ AIDS prevention programs have the difficult goal of introducing and motivating the change to safer sex. It is a complicated task which requires an appreciation of both intergenerational norms and intragenerational trends, individual decision-making, and the sequencing of partner interactions. This chapter suggests the impact of time at both macro- and microlevels.

At the societal and community level, sexual behaviour is often the outcome of past customs and traditions rather than the result of a decision based on the risk of contracting AIDS. The advice to have protected sex runs counter to powerful traditional values associated with fertility and procreation, rites of passage to adulthood, religious values and the exchange of semen.

The predominance of the medical model (see Guizzardi, *et al.*, Chapter 9) and insensitivity to cultural norms has plagued prevention efforts. There are many examples where customs clash with current prevention efforts. Programs have attempted to provide condoms to women and men whose status is highly related to procreation or where the meaning of intimacy is historically linked with the exchange of semen. Often programs have run into resistance from clergy who have historically forbidden artificial contraception. Even when the consequences of AIDS are well known these cultural barriers are difficult to overcome.

It is usually easier to incorporate long-held values into prevention programs than to present a new behaviour that contradicts past customs and beliefs. Where programs confront long-held values, interventions at the policy and community level increase the likelihood of success. Where the program depends on a lack of discrimination against those with HIV, policies that attack the roots of discrimination will have a positive effect on lowering the rate of HIV infection. For example, a frequent prevention strategy is empowering women in societies that have traditionally given them no power. This approach will be more successful if women are educated, organized, have the means to acquire income and property, and face less discrimination.

Current trends and events often provide the stimulus to challenge long-held values and norms. Traditional sexual values have changed due to scientific discoveries such as the pill, and social upheavals such as disease, war, urban violence and famine. For example, the political and social instability in the former Soviet Union has created conditions which contribute to the spread of HIV. Given current trends, there are likely to be exploding epidemics among the homosexual populations in Eastern Europe as newly expressed sexual freedoms contribute to risky sexual behaviour for HIV infection. Regional wars and civil wars, such as in the former Yugoslavia, have caused forced migration and widespread sexual abuse for the general population. Some immigrants find that sex work provides a means to survive and often lack the knowledge, access to condoms, or self-efficacy to engage in safer sex. Programs directed at the community level which decrease poverty assure the human rights of immigrants, moderate violence, and provide economic opportunity will have an impact on reducing the threat of HIV infection.

The HIV epidemic itself has served as a catalyst to change sexual norms. However, the belief that the epidemic is self-regulating once persons are aware of others with AIDS has proven false, and there is evidence that continued prevention in the tail of the epidemic is necessary to maintain the adoption of safer sexual practices. There is no doubt that communities have changed their sexual behaviour because of AIDS. Unfortunately, many changes have not been effective and many are based on misperceptions about the causes of HIV transmission and a lack of awareness of the long lag between infection and manifestation of AIDS.

One great challenge for HIV prevention is impressing on communities the long-term consequences of AIDS. Effective early action when the epidemic first appears in a community could reduce its impact. Unfortunately, most communities and governments respond late in the HIV epidemic. Given the time lag between HIV infection and AIDS, by the time AIDS becomes a public health issue, the HIV epidemic is usually well established in the community.

For individuals their time frame for making decisions about sexual behaviour is critical to understanding their behaviour. HIV/AIDS prevention programs often fail because they assume that the life and death consequences of HIV infection will be the most important factors in deciding about sexual behaviour. That is a wrong assumption. Many find more immediate gains from social acceptance, love, financial gain, or other rewards that hold a far greater value than some distant chance of dying from AIDS. In addition, individuals usually underestimate their own risk of HIV. Targeting interventions in the domain of greatest concern to an individual is likely to be more successful than repeating messages about the long-term consequences of HIV. For example, more persons will adopt safer sex if it is associated with eroticism, love, intimacy and concern for partners than only emphasizing the distant deadly consequences of AIDS.

The same information may be seen quite differently for individuals in different stages of the decision-making process. Timing of information may be more important than the information itself. For many, the domain of AIDS is outside their concern, and despite the prevention program, they are not likely to process any of the information. Others may be in a stage where they are trying to assess their own risk. At this stage having the tools to assess their own risk accurately is important. Still others may be ready to make a commitment to safer sex. For them, social support, a sense of self-efficacy and enjoying safer sex are likely to be very important. Last, for those who have adopted safer sex, reinforcement of positive attitudes, social support and strategies to adopt safer sex in their relationship are important in helping them to maintain safer sex.

Individuals may also be at different times in their life cycle. Prevention programs should be designed for critical situations that occur in each life cycle phase. Those who are defining their sexual identity should have the information and skills to defer the initiation of sexual intercourse or use of safer sex. As partnerships form, partner negotiation skills become essential. Once in a relationship, strategies for safer sex in maintaining a relationship are needed. The task is to determine what are the most appropriate messages for individuals and partners in each of these phases and find channels of communication used by individuals and partners in each of the phases. For the individual, then, understanding the cost and benefits of unsafe and safer sex, the timing in the decision-making process and the timing of their life cycle are each important considerations in developing HIV-prevention programs. But often the individual is not the best focus for prevention programs.

Sex occurs between partners, and how they come to agree upon safer or unsafe sex may be largely a function of their interaction. Partners who do not engage in safer sex should be taught to communicate about safer sex and practice communication skills with their partners. The goals of a prevention program should be to change the norm of a community where safer sex is viewed as an expression of concern and love rather than one of infidelity or lack of trust. Until that time, partners will have to learn how to introduce safer sex into their relationships.

In most societies love appears to be an obstacle to safer sex. Partners who do start with safer sex often change to unprotected sex as the need for closeness increases. After a few episodes of intercourse unprotected sex is frequently viewed by the partners as an expression of trust and a way to feel closer to each other. Prevention programs, often targeted towards casual sex, have been deficient in developing strategies for partners in love.

Like individuals who go through stages, couples may also pass through stages in their relationships. Understanding the timing of the seduction, familiarity and denouncement stages will provide some insight into different prevention programs for each stage. The idea here is to design specific prevention programs for risk behaviour common in the different stages. This would be a substantial change from the more frequent strategy of targeting groups based on stable social or behavioural attributes (such as poverty or drug use). For example, many programs today are directed towards younger individuals because they are more likely to be in the seduction stage and have a high likelihood of multiple partners. However, even more mature partners in the denouncement stage in one relationship may also be in the seduction stage in another relationship. They and their partners are particularly at risk because they are likely to engage in unsafe sex during their dissolving relationship and in their new relationships. Specific programs could be implemented at venues where they meet, such as clubs or singles bars, or through health care professionals such as marriage guidance counselors. Other gaps in prevention programs might become clearer if those designing programs thought more in terms of time than demographics.

While not exhaustive, this last section shows that taking account of time is a necessary part of any HIV-prevention program. Typically, intergenerational values have been underestimated. Equally important is understanding the reasons for current trends and styles related to unsafe behaviour. Where the causes of unsafe sex are economic need, illiteracy or violence, action at the community level may be more effective than programs which inform individuals. At the individual level information about the proximate needs and the stage of their decision-making can be used to develop effective prevention programs. However, sex occurs between partners and is influenced by peer norms. Understanding the sequencing of partner and peer interactions may provide the key to developing HIV/AIDS prevention programs which successfully motivate persons to engage in safer sex.

Notes

1 *Community* is used throughout the text to refer to populations bound by some common self-identifying geographic and psychosocial trait. While HIV/AIDS prevention programs are often planned at a national level, the most effective programs speak to the needs of specific communities effected by the epidemic.
2 *Unsafe sex* in this text refers to sex without a condom where the HIV status of the partner is not known for certain or one partner is seropositive.

References

ABRAMSON, P. and HERDT, G. (1990) 'The assessment of sexual practices relevant to the transmission of AIDS: A global perspective', *Journal of Sex Research*, **27**, pp. 215–32.
AGRAFIOTIS, D. (1990) 'Knowledge, attitudes, beliefs and practices in relation to HIV

infection and AIDS: The case of the city of Athens (Greece)', unpublished report, Athens: Athens School of Public Health, Department of Sociology.

ALBERT, E. (1988) 'Illness and/or deviance: The response of the press to AIDS', in FELDMAN, D. and JOHNSON, T.M. *Social Dimensions of AIDS: Methods and Theory*, New York: Praeger.

ANKRAH, E. (1990) 'Women and AIDS in Africa: Socio-cultural issues of empowerment', paper presented at AIDS and Reproductive Health: Agenda for Research and Action, unpublished paper, Ballogio, Italy, November.

ATTIAS-DONFUT, C. (1988) *Sociologie des générations*, Paris: Presses universitaires de France.

BANDURA, A. (1977a) 'Self-efficacy: Towards a unifying theory of behavioural change', *Psychological Review*, **84**, pp. 191–215.

BANDURA, A. (1977b) *Social Learning Theory*, Englewood Cliffs, NJ: Prentice Hall.

BANDURA, A. (1988) 'Perceived self-efficacy in the exercise of control over AIDS infection', in BLUMENTHAL, A., EICHLER, G., WEISMANN, *et al.* (Eds) *Women and AIDS*, Washington, DC: American Psychiatric Press.

BOER, D., KOK, G., HOSPERS, H. and GERARDS, F. (1991) 'Health education strategies for the attributional retraining and self-efficacy improvement', *Health Education Research*, **6** (2), pp. 239–48.

BROWN, P. (1992) 'AIDS in the media', in MANN, J., TARANTOLA, D. and NETTER, T. (Eds) *AIDS in the World*, Cambridge, MA: Harvard University Press, pp. 720–32.

BYE, L. (1987) 'A report on designing an effective AIDS prevention campaign strategy for San Francisco: Results of the 2nd probability sample of the urban gay male community', San Francisco, CA: AIDS Foundation.

CARRIER, J., MAGANA, M. and RAUL, J. (1991) 'Use of ethnosexual data on men of Mexican origin for HIV/AIDS prevention programs', *Journal of Sex Research*, **28**, pp. 189–201.

CASADONTE, P., JARLAIS, D., FRIEDMAN, S. and ROSTROSEN, J. (1990) 'Psychological and behavioral impact among IDUs of learning HIV-test results', *International Journal of Addiction*, **25** (4), pp. 409–26.

CATANIA, J., KEGELES, S. and COATES, T. (1990) 'Towards an understanding of risk behaviour: An AIDS risk reduction model (ARRM)', *Health Education Quarterly*, **17**, pp. 53–72.

CLIFT, S. and STEARS, D. (1991) 'Moral perspectives and safer sex practice: Two themes in teaching about HIV and AIDS in secondary schools', in AGGLETON, P., HART, G. and DAVIS, P. (Eds) *AIDS: Responses, Interventions and Care*, London: Falmer Press, pp. 169–89.

COHEN, M. (1991) 'Changing to safer sex: Personality, logic and habit', in AGGLETON, P., HART, G. and DAVIS, P. (Eds) *AIDS: Responses Interventions and Care*, London: Falmer Press, pp. 19–41.

COHEN, M. (1992) 'The global response: Prevention', in MANN, J., TARANTOLA, D. and NETTER, T. (Eds) *AIDS in the World*, Cambridge, MA: Harvard University Press, pp. 325–448.

COHEN, M. and CHWALOW, J. (1993) 'Using theoretical frameworks to evaluate the effectiveness of HIV prevention programs: Determining factors related to sexual behavior change by stages of the HIV epidemic', unpublished, Inserm U 21, Paris.

COHEN, M., TRANATOLA, D., NETTER, T., CASE, P. and MANN, J. (1992) 'Worldwide response to HIV prevention', presentation at the 8th International Conference on AIDS/III Std, World Congress, Amsterdam: July.

CONNELL, R.W., CRAWFORD, G., DOWSETT, G., KIPPAX, S., CENT, V., RODDEN, P., BOOCTER, D., BERG, R. and WATSON, L. (1989) 'Unsafe anal sexual practice among homosexual men', NSW, Australia: Macquarie University, pp. 1–34.

CONNELL, R., CRAWFORD, J., KIPPAX, S. and DOWSETT, G., *et al.* (1988) 'Facing the epidemic: Changes in the sexual and social lives of gay and bisexual men in response to the AIDS crisis', Report 3, NSW, Australia: Macquarie University.

CONNELL, R., DOWSETT, G., and RODDEN, P. (1991) 'Social class, gay men and AIDS prevention', *Australian Journal of Public Health*, **15** (3), pp. 178–89.

DESJARLAIS, D. and FRIEDMAN, S. (1989) 'An overview of AIDS among IDUs/epidemiology, natural history and prevention', Stricting Drug Symposium, Amsterdam.

DE VRIES, H., DIJKSTRA, M. and KUHLMAN, P. (1988) 'Self-efficacy: The third factor besides attitude and subjective norm as a predictor of behavioral intentions', *Health Education Research*, **3** (3), pp. 273–82.

DE WIT, J., VROOME, E., SANDFORT, T., VAN GRIENSVEN, G., *et al.* (1991) 'Increase in the incidence of HIV infections in relation to higher levels of unsafe sexual behavior, in a cohort of homosexual men in Amsterdam', Utrecht, Netherlands: University of Utrecht, Department of Gay and Lesbian Studies.

DWYER, D., HOWARD, R., DOWNIE, J. and CUNNINGHAM, A.N., *et al.* (1988) 'The "grim reaper" campaign', *Medical Journal of Australia*, **149**, pp. 49–50.

FRANK, O. (1992) 'Sexual behaviour and disease transmission in Sub-Saharan Africa: Past trends and future prospects', in DYSON, T. (Ed.) *Sexual Behaviour and Networking: Anthropological and Socio-Cultural Studies on the Transmission of HIV*, Liège: Derouaux, Ordina Editions, pp. 89–108.

FRAZER, I.M., MALCOLM, M., HAY, I. and NORTH, P. (1988) 'Influence of HIV antibody testing on sexual behaviour in a "high-risk" population from a "low-risk" city', *Medical Journal of Australia*, **149**, pp. 365–8.

FRIEDMAN, S., LEVINE, M. and SIEGEL, K. (1986) 'AIDS: The formulation of a sociological perspective', Chicago, IL: Society for the Study of Social Problems, pp. 1–23.

FRUTCHEY, C. (1989) 'The role of community based organizations in AIDS and STD prevention', in PAALMAN, M. (Ed.) *Promoting Safer Sex*, Amsterdam: Swets and Zeitlinger, pp. 81–92.

FULLILOVE, M. (1992) 'Trading sex for drugs', in MANN, J., TARANTOLA, D. and NETTER, T. (Eds), *AIDS in the World*, Cambridge, MA: Harvard University Press, p. 377.

GRAY, J. (1985) 'Growing yams and men: An interpretation of Kimam male ritualized homosexual behavior', *Journal of Homosexual Behavior Special Issue: Anthropology of Homosexual Behavior*, **11** (3–4), pp. 55–68.

HARDY, D. (1988) 'Cultural practices contributing to the transmission of human immunodeficiency virus in Africa', in KOCH-WESER, D. and VANDERSCHMIDT, H. (Eds) *The Heterosexual Transmission of AIDS in Africa*, Cambridge, MA: ABT Books, pp. 255–64.

Mitchell Cohen and Michel Hubert

HEIDER, F. (1958) *The Psychology of Interpersonal Relations*, New York: John Wiley.

HERZLICH, C. and PIERRET, J. (1989) 'The construction of a social phenomenon: AIDS in the French press', *Social Science Medicine*, **28** (11), pp. 1235–42.

HERDT, G. (1982) 'Fetish and fantasy in Sambian initiation', in HERDT, G. (Eds) *Ritual of Manhood: Male Initiation in New Guinea*, Berkeley, CA: University of California Press.

HERGENHAHN, B.R. (1982) *An Introduction to Theories of Learning*, Englewood Cliffs, NJ: Prentice-Hall Inc.

HESSOL, N., LIFTON, A., O'MALLEY, P., DOLL, L. *et al.* (1989) 'Prevalence, incidence, and progression of HIV infection in homosexual and bisexual men in hepatitis B. vaccine trials, 1987–1988', *American Journal of Epidemiology*, **130** (6), pp. 1167–1175.

HUBERT, M. and MARQUET, J. (Coordonnateurs), DELCHAMBRE, J.-P., PETO, D., SCHAUT, C. and VAN CAMPENHOUDT, L. (1993) 'Comportements sexuels et réactions au risque du Sida en Belgique', Brussels: Centre d'études sociologiques, Facultés universitaires Saint-Louis.

HUGGINS, J., ELMAN, N., BAKER, C., FORRESTER, R., *et al.* (1991) 'Affective and behavioural responses of gay and bisexual men to HIV antibody testing', *Social Work*, **36**, pp. 61–6.

HUNT, A. and DAVIES, P. (1991) 'What is a sexual encounter?', in AGGLETON, P., HART, G. and DAVIES, P. (Eds) *AIDS: Response Interventions and Care*, London: Falmer Press, pp. 43–52.

JOHNSON, A., WADSWORTH, J., WELLINGS, K., BRADSHAW, S. and FIELD, J. (1992) 'Sexual lifestyles and HIV risk', *Nature*, **3**, pp. 410–12.

JOHNSON, A., WADSWORTH, J., WELLINGS, K. and FIELD, J. (1994) *Sexual Attitudes and Lifestyles*, London: Blackwell Scientific Publications.

KAPLAN, M. (1990) 'AIDS and the psycho-social discipines: The social control of "Dangerous" behaviour', *Journal of Mind and Behaviour*, **11**, pp. 337–52.

KELLY, J., ST. LAWRENCE, J., BRASFIELD, T. and HOOD, H. (1989) 'Group interventions to reduce AIDS risk behaviours in gay men: Applications of behavioural principles', in MAYS, V., ALBEE, G. and SCHNEIDER, S. (Eds) *Primary Prevention of AIDS*, London: Sage, pp. 225–41.

KELLY, J., LAWRENCE, J., BRASFIELD, T., STEVENSON, Y., DIAZ, Y. and HAUTH, A. (1990) 'AIDS risk behaviour patterns among gay men in small southern cities', *American Journal of Public Health*, **80**, pp. 416–18.

KIPPAX, S., CRAWFORD, C., CONNELL, R. and DOWSETT, G. (1990) 'The importance of gay community in the prevention of HIV transmission', *Social Aspects of the Prevention of AIDS*, a, 7, pp. 1–48.

KOHLBERG, L. (1983) *Moral Stages*, New York: Karger.

LALLEMANT, M., LALLEMENT-LE COEUR, S., CHEYNIER, D., NZINGOULA, S., JOURDAIN, G., SINET, M., DAZZA, M. and LAROUZE, B. (1992) 'Characteristics associated with HIV-1 infection in pregnant women in Brazzaville, Congo', *AIDS*, **5** (3), pp. 279–85.

LAUMANN, E., GAGNON, J., MICHAEL, R. and MICHAELS, S. (1994) *The Social Organization of Sexuality: Sexual Practices in the United States.* Chicago, IL: University of Chicago Press.

LENNEER-AXELSON, B. (1988) 'Sexuality in the shadow of AIDS: Some reflections on the future', presentation at The 4th International Conference on AIDS, Stockholm: June.

McCUSKER, J., STODDARD, A., ZAPKA, J., ZORN, J. and MAYER, K. (1989a) 'Predictors of AIDS-preventive behaviour among homosexually active men: A longitudinal study', *AIDS*, **3**, pp. 443–8.

McCUSKER, J., ZAPKA, J., STODDARD, A. and MAYER, K. (1989b) 'Responses to the AIDS epidemic among homosexually active men: Factors associated with preventive behaviour', *Patient Education and Counseling*, **13**, pp. 15–30.

McGUIRE, W. (1991) 'Using guiding-idea theories of the person to develop educational campaigns against drug abuse and other health-threatening behaviour', *Health Education Research*, **6**, pp. 173–84.

MARTIN, J. (1986) 'AIDS risk reduction recommendations and sexual behaviour patterns among gay men: A multifactorial categorical approach to assessing change', *Health Education Quarterly*, **13**, pp. 347–58.

MARTIN, J., DEAN, L., BARCIA, M. and HALL, W. (1989) 'The impact of AIDS on a gay community: Changes in sexual behaviour, substance use and mental health', *American Journal of Community Psychology*, **17**, pp. 269–93.

MEMON, A. (1991) 'Perceptions of the AIDS vulnerability: The role of attributions and social context', in AGGLETON, P., HART, P. and DAVIS, P. (Eds) *AIDS: Responses, Interventions and Care*, London: Falmer Press, pp. 157–68.

MOATTI, J.-P. and POLLAK, M. (1990) 'Hiv risk perception and determinants of sexual behaviour', in HUBERT, M. (Ed.) *Sexual Behaviour and Risks of Hiv Infection: Proceedings of an International Workshop Supported by the European Communities*, Brussels: Publications des Facultés universitaires Saint-Louis, Collection Travaux et Recherches.

MONTGOMERY, S., JOSEPH, J., BECKER, M., OSTROW, D., KESSLER, R., KIRSCHT, J. (1989) 'The health belief model in understanding compliance with preventive recommendations for AIDS: How useful?', *AIDS Education and Prevention*, **1**, pp. 303–23.

NGUMA, J. (1992) 'Early perceptions and misperceptions about AIDS in Tanzania', in MANN, J., TARANTOLA, D. and NETTER, T. (Eds) *AIDS in the World*, Cambridge, MA: Harvard University Press, pp. 332–3.

O'MALLEY, J. (1992) 'AIDS service organizations in transition', in MANN, J., TARANTOLA, D. and NETTER, T. (Eds) *AIDS in the World*, Cambridge, MA: Harvard University Press, pp. 774–87.

PARKER, R. and TAWIL, O. (1991) 'Bisexual behaviour and HIV transmission in Latin America', in TIELMAN, R., CARBALLO, M., HENDRIKS, A. (Eds) *Bisexuality and HIV/AIDS*, Buffalo, NY: Prometheus Books, pp. 59–64.

PETO, D., REMY, J., VAN CAMPENHOUDT, L. and HUBERT, M. (1992) *Sida. L'amour face à la peur. Modes d'adaptation au risque du Sida dans les relations hétérosexuelles*, Paris: L'Harmattan, Collection Logiques Sociales.

POLLAK, M. (1991) 'Assessing prevention for men having sex with men', European Concerted Action on Assessment of AIDS/HIV Prevention, Lausanne: Institut de médecine sociale et préventive. Cahiers de recherches et de documentation, **75**.

PRIEUR, A. (1990) 'Norwegian gay men: Reasons for continued practice of unsafe sex', *AIDS Education and Prevention*, **2**, pp. 109–15.

PROCHAZKA, I. (1994) 'The perception of HIV-risk among Czech gay men', presented at AIDS in Europe: The Behavioural Aspect, Berlin: September 26–29.

ROBERT, B. and ROSSER, S. (1990) 'Evaluation of the efficacy of AIDS education interventions for homosexually active men', *Health Education Research*, **5**, pp. 299–308.

ROSENSTOCK, I., STRECHER, V. and BECKER, M. (1988) 'Social learning theory and the health belief model', *Health Education Quarterly*, **15**, pp. 175–83.

SHEEHY, G. (1976) *Passages*, New York: Dalton.

SPIRA, A., BAJOS, N. et le Groupe ACSF (1993) *Les Comportements sexuels en France*, Paris: La Documentation Française, Collection des Rapports Officiels.

STALL, R., COHEN, M., DOWSETT, G., VAN GRIENSVEN G., HART, G. and KELLY (1992) 'Maintenance of HIV risk reduction among gay-identified men', in MANN, J., TARANTOLA, D. and NETTER, T. (Eds) *AIDS in the World*, Cambridge, MA: Harvard University Press, pp. 653–67.

STALL, R. and PAUL, J. (1989) 'Changes in the sexual risk for infection with the HIV virus among gay and bisexual men in San Francisco', Consultation on Risk Reduction among Gay and Bisexual Men, Geneva, May.

TAYLOR, C. (1990) 'Condoms and cosmology: The fractal person and sexual risk in Rwanda', *Social Science Medicine*, **30**, pp. 1023–8.

TOMASEVSKI, K. (1992) 'AIDS and human rights', in MANN, J., TARANTOLA, D. and NETTER, T. (Eds) *AIDS in the World*, Cambridge, MA: Harvard University Press, pp. 537–73.

VALDISERRI, R. (1989) *Preventing AIDS: The Design of Effective Programs*, New Brunswick, NJ: Rutgers University.

VAN GRIENSVEN, G., VROOME, E. and TIELMAN, R. (1988) 'Impact of antibody testing on changes in sexual behavior among homosexual men in the Netherlands', *American Journal of Public Health*, **78**, pp. 1575–77.

VAN ZESSEN, G. and SANDFORT, T. (1991) *Seksualiteit in Nederland; Seksueel Gedrag, Risico en Preventie van AIDS*, Amsterdam/Lisse: Swets & Zeitlinger.

WEINSTEIN, N. (1989) 'Perceptions of personal susceptibility to harm', in MAYS, V., ALBEE, G. and SCHNEIDER, S. (Eds) *Primary Prevention of AIDS*, London: Sage Publications, pp. 142–67.

WEISMAN, C., NATHANSON, C., ENSMINGER, M., TEITELBAUM, M. *et al.* (1989) 'AIDS knowledge, perceived risk and prevention among adolescent clients of a family planning clinic', *Family Planning Perspectives*, **21**, pp. 213–17.

WELLINGS, K. (1991) 'Netherlands: Country Report', European Concerted Action on Assessment of HIV/AIDS Prevention, London.

Chapter 12

Norms of Relationship and Normative Tensions

Gustavo Guizzardi

The Nature of the Problem

It must be recognized that the advent of the HIV infection has given rise to a new situation, namely, the reappearance of explicit normativization as regards sexual behaviour. Whereas, for a relatively brief period, sexuality was simply a private action without normativization, it now belongs markedly to the public sphere. We are witnessing the growth of very detailed and explicit information about HIV and AIDS that includes how it originated, how it is transmitted, who may be infected and what the future holds. Most of all, what we have before us is the elaboration and codification of *prescriptive* collective norms regarding the private life of each and every individual, both generally (how concerned we should be, how we should behave towards those infected, etc.), and more intimately (how we should behave in our sex lives). This normativization has certain specific features. Its *form* is a message that is present and visible, especially in the mass communication media.

The *content* upon which the norms are constructed consists of at least two elements. The first is partly new and apparently very simple: 'Sexual behaviour should conform to the technical norms of safer sex.' There is no explicit reference to the values which should underlie such behaviour or to the way it is judged. In fact, the norms of safer sex may appear highly tolerant and suggest that any objective pursued through sexuality is both acceptable and accepted. The message seems minimal: 'Behave as you usually do but modify your actions in this one small detail by using the techniques of safer sex.' This technical micro-modification appears capable of producing great changes without altering the behavioural aims and preferences of the individual. The second component of sexual normativity refers instead to those older coercive norms legitimated within a vast framework of values. We are concerned here with the norms which govern the duty of fidelity within the stable couple, chastity and so on. The duty contained in the norm is, if anything, presented no longer (or not only) as behaviour stemming from values above the level of the individual, but rather as common sense advice valid for the present circumstances in line with the old rules of conduct.

Every system of norms requires legitimation. In this case, there is a two-phase process. The first process is the need for immediate legitimation, and the second the need for a basic legitimation of the norms. The technical micro-normativity briefly outlined finds its immediate legitimation by referring to a policy of prevention, the only policy which can be pursued in the short and medium term and 'that has to aim at modifying particular patterns of sexual behaviour that have been identified as the main channels for transmitting the virus' (Ahlemeyer and Ludwig, Chapter 2). The choice of this path is not a neutral one. The identification of bio-medical factors (a virus or a series of viruses) as the cause of the AIDS epidemic leads to the pinpointing of the source, or rather the main source, for legitimizing the norms. This source is authoritarian in nature: the authority of particular technical specialists with official functions within the medical field. This change tends to lessen the authority of the traditional experts in ethics and values and shift authority within the medical field from physicians to specialists in bio-medicine and bio-engineering. The creation of a new source of legitimacy is strengthened by the contingent but significant dramatization of the time and place of the epidemic's effects. The site of the drama is no longer restricted to the small circle of affected people, but has shifted to the entire community. The time available is emphasized as very short and, in any case, wholly inadequate.

This extreme dramatization is a central feature of the phenomenon. Its main effect is that we end up identifying a fundamental – no longer transient – principle for legitimizing the message and actions, in other words the norms themselves. The total dramatization of time (we must act immediately), the size of the phenomenon (the epidemic concerns us all) and, lastly, the object itself (AIDS is fatal) lead to the pinpointing of a legitimizing criterion presented as being universally shared even in complex and fragmented societies such as those of the West. This criterion is a variation on the traditional principle of the common good: 'No matter how individually separate we are and no matter how much we continue to pursue our private, sometimes opposing aims, we must all unite in the primary and irremissible objective of saving the entire community.' This type of legitimation is therefore founded on the universal value of the common good, a value that has reappeared and is again valid in a now fully technological age.

The logic of *limited technical normativity*, in its apparent simplicity, seems, at least in part, to underpin this implicit value system. Indeed, normativization in the sexual field, denoted as safer sex, may be interpreted as conforming to the value that the collective benefit to everybody of safer sex is so great that the disadvantages for the individual are of minor importance, or even individuals should be reasonable and subordinate their temporary private benefit to the lasting public one. Thus, the preventive message, so tolerant in form, would appear to be confirmed as rational and reasonable once again. However, all the research shows that, at various levels and in different aspects, these particular preventive norms are not followed (for an articulate, detailed synthesis, see Pryor and Reeder, 1993). This observation gives rise to a series of problems, the first of which is pragmatic in nature. As Gerrard, *et al.* (1993) state, 'If convincing people that they are at risk for HIV infection does not alter their sexual behaviour, then what possibly could?'

Another problem emerges at a theoretical level. One question asked by Ahlemeyer and Ludwig – What is 'the contribution of the norm concept to improving practical preventive effort?' – goes to the heart of the matter. But most of all, we should ask ourselves if sexual behaviour can be changed through normativization. As Ahlemeyer and Ludwig ask, 'the question arises whether HIV preventive efforts could use normative means in order to bring about the desired change in sexual behaviour.' In addition, what type of normativization is involved? Who is capable of establishing the norms and who is able to change them?

Sexual Normativity and Social Normativity: The Dyadic System and its Autonomy

The chapters which constitute this volume render these questions even more pressing because they are based on research and delve further into the specific aspects of sexual relations in couples. In various ways they support the view that the rules of sexual normativity are separate from those of social normativity. What type of separation concerns us here? Citing Luhmann, Ahlemeyer says that the basic system is 'the interactive system between two intimate partners', which forms 'a dyadic system of intimate communication'. It is a system with three main features:

- it is independent of the environment;
- it constantly produces and reproduces its constituent elements (the principle of *autopoiesis*); and
- it possesses a dynamic that is endogenously produced by the dyad.

However autonomous, autopoietic, endogenous and restless it may be, the system is structured, for functional requirements, according to its own establishing logic. This is to limit the great complexity of facts and solutions available to the actors and reduce the super-abundance of possibilities that ceaselessly appear and disappear. In this sense we may speak of norms within and belonging to the dyadic system of intimate communication. According to Ahlemeyer, 'norms are a particular form of the structure of social systems;

expectations which are upheld even after their disappointment.' In this interpretative model the existence of norms is essential, since 'the main function of norms is to help solving problems of continuity, warding off the constant threat of collapse which is posed by everyday reality.' We may even say that the dyadic system of intimate communication is one in which the norms appear even more necessary since there is not 'a sphere where expectations are as risky and susceptible to disappointment as in sexuality.'

We have here a very interesting aspect, the presence of tension between the two poles: autopoiesis, i.e., the continual production of liberty, on the one hand, and normativization, i.e., strict regulation, on the other. The tension between the two resolves into the system's own *autopoietic normativization*. The dyadic system would appear to be totally autonomous. However, there are opportunities for permeation with the norms of the environment. Indeed the presence of norms autonomously generated by the dyad does not mean that the dyad can establish any norm whatever for itself. It might maintain that it could do so, regard itself as autopoietic, but could equally not be so due to the contents of the norms established. The dyad is, in fact, an autonomous communication system, but its autonomy lies in the communication, not necessarily in the content communicated.

This seems to be the pathway along which, according to Ahlemeyer's model, the external norms enter the intimate system, and also through which the intimate system can relate to the environment: 'Norms pose requirements of participation.' Even research into sexual behaviour shows that relationships hinge on trust between the partners, and this means that a relationship modality is stressed irrespective of its content; on the one hand, there is autopoiesis but, on the other, there is a way open from the dyadic system to the environment.

At a system level, we may note how social norms come into play by means of the structuring of the forms of communicative sexual systems available in a society (Ahlemeyer points out four). However, other limitations regarding normativization are also present. In Ahlemeyer's model, for example, the erotic system is dyadic and the type of erotic communication is heterosexual. This means that there are elements which socially normativize the communication itself, by indicating, for example, the content suitable or that particular relational structure. All this shows that while there is pressure from the social system on the dyadic one, that the contrary, i.e., the pressure of the dyadic system of intimate communication on other systems, is also true. There is, in any case, a fixed course in the model – the concrete intervention of social actors.

Clearly the system of intimate communication does not focus on the individuals who take part in it but on the communication itself. It is also true that, being autopoietic, the system creates a radical rift between erotic reality and everyday life. However, it is equally clear that the system is made up of individuals who, after all, are the only ones who give content to the system itself and who experience both the sphere of everyday life and the system of erotic reality. They, therefore, are the carriers of the relations between the complex system and that of intimate communication, general social norms and the specific norms of the sexuality system. In any case, the model demonstrates one important point – the system of intimate communication cannot be passed over. Normative indications from outside must cross the barrier which consists of the norms which the dyadic system has created, and must become relevant to the dyadic system. This they do to the extent that they are constituted within the system.

Socialization, Shared Reality, Point of Reference

Ludwig's position on norms is somewhat different. First, she focuses more on the individual and his or her cognitive aspects. Second, she attributes a very different meaning to the concept of the norm. There is an inter-individual social site, where values, representations of collective reference and norms are created, and there also exists a process by which the results of this intense collective activity become the property of the individual.

The key point is the process of socialization, i.e., the way in which an individual becomes a member of a group, shares a culture and participates in a reality shared by others. At this key point, norms – defined as *prescriptive standards* (how people should behave) – come into play. They are acquired through socialization and considered among the most significant aspects of culture. According to her interpretation norms acquire a central and necessary role. 'One of their most important functions is to offer a point of reference with the help of which evaluations and judgments are made.' It should be noted that by norm she, unlike Ahlemeyer, intends its content; moreover, respect for the norm becomes very important in order for the individual to be part of the group, i.e., to accede to the fundamental characteristic of the individual which is sociality, i.e., the wish to be accepted by the others. Thus, talk of norms has a dual meaning – socially produced behaviour rules (prescriptive standards of behaviour), and also prescriptive rules valid for the individual. However, society and the individual do not occupy symmetrical positions. Society seems free to provide the contents of the norms, whereas the individual is not free to change them, or enjoys only a limited freedom to do so. Perhaps in the field of sexuality this tension between individual autonomy and social regulation is greater since, on the one hand, the domains of sexual interaction are among the most strictly socially regulated, but on the other, 'they also belong to the most private sphere, in which partners are allowed, to some extent, to define their own rules.'

It seems more difficult to understand where the relative autonomy in the sexual sphere lies with respect to the norms, particularly when the concept of norm also becomes a pattern which defines normality, determines

Gustavo Guizzardi

what is normal and what is abnormal or pathological. Thus normativization is viewed in a strong, heteronomous sense with respect to the individual or group. The problem posed at the beginning, why the norms on safe sex are not followed, appears here more serious, since one would expect the opposite, i.e., that they be followed. The answer which might emerge from this model may refer, on the one hand, to relative freedom in private life. We may, on the other hand, be in a period of transition; a somewhat lengthy period of time is required for the norms produced at a social level to be introduced into the socialization apparatus, internalized and accepted. Or does the key mechanism perhaps lie within the reference group and, more precisely, in the others by whom we wish to be accepted?

The Individual, the Network and My Other Self

The two previous models set aside the complexity of the social environment; one because it centres on the autonomy of the dyadic system (Ahlemeyer), and the other because it hypothesizes in fact that the complex society is sufficiently compact to provide a unitary and consistent socialization in its various sectors. But what happens in the opposite and more frequent situation? What happens when the set of norms is not consistent and may even be contradictory; when the norms are highly sectoral, so that there are semi-structured spheres, others without norms, and yet others which are strictly regulated? In this situation, both individuals and groups are faced with a vast plurality of inconsistent norms which are not equally binding and are strict and far-reaching to varying degrees.

The model put forward by Ferrand and Snijders (Chapter 1) seems to be placed within a social structure closer to this situation and features accentuated pluralism. Their response to the problem of the efficacy of social norms regarding safer sex is totally negative. They maintain that 'collective norms are not prescribed by medical or public health agencies, but by groups and networks on the basis of some collective interest in their application'. The central point of the hypothesis is given by two basic choices that have to be made. The first has to do with the level of social aggregation which they feel is significant, i.e., the networks in which the individual participates, interpersonal relations and not individual behaviour. The second is the criterion which governs the individual's choice. This, according to Coleman's theory, is rationality. Thus, norms exist and are even accentuated, but they are bound to networks and, what is more, conditioned by them. The norm is a specific right of control over the individual's behaviour, and being so it is above the others, i.e., the members of the network.

In this model, therefore, the principle of the heteronomy of the individual is strong, but it is ascribed to the network and not the whole of society. In fact the network itself is specified by the norms which are in force within it and also has the function of being 'the carrier of norms about behaviour' (Chapter 1). Even in this hypothesis, however, we find tension between the individual and the network. First, the individual is (relatively) free to belong to or choose the network, and this freedom is increased by the plurality of existing networks – both homogeneous and heterogeneous – and their unity or otherwise in offering norms. Second, the individual may withdraw from the control of others by hiding those parts of his behaviour which would be disapproved of or by clearly demonstrating only those approved of.

Moreover, there is a second tension between the individual and the network; the individual is, at the same time, both himself and one of the others, with regard to the participants in the network. In this second role he has to apply the sanctions if someone does not follow the norms. This gives rise to a third form of tension – the individual runs the risk of being pushed aside if he acts alone and therefore to leave the network if he or she enforces the norms too strictly. Or, something which the authors do not state explicitly, the individual/enforcer runs the risk of breaking up the network itself.

Thus we arrive at the dual nature of this model; while the individual's principle is basically rational, that which governs the aggregation of individuals is not. The individual's will to belong to a network, pursued as the main, independent factor, is due to a desire to socialize and share goals and affections. The tension lies in the dual role of the others (and therefore of each to the rest) who are at the same time significant others and controlling others. In the first case the norm – sticking to the norm and maintaining that others should stick to it – gives pleasure (that of being approved of and approving); in the second it is the vehicle for conflict (that of being disapproved of and disapproving).

The problem is to see how long this equilibrium, which at a psychological level appears in the tension between trust and suspicion, will last. The authors point out that this is a particularly serious aspect for sexuality (the individual respects neither the norm nor specific rational interest when driven by pleasure) and maintain that it is the others who should undertake to apply sanctions, and recall the rationality of the behaviour. 'In love relations, because love is love, sexual partners are not necessarily interested by their own interest, but others as alters, in a more detached and cool appreciation of what is going on, are interested in the health of their friends' (Chapter 9).

Apparently, we need to play down the normative and rational component and stress the participatory one, that is, place the emphasis on friendship rather than the norm. The other possibility is to stress the disparity of positions within the network. Thus, the significant others acquire a position of power over the individual, not so much directly as indirectly, in the field of emotions. It is emotionally very costly to change one's point of reference, withdraw from the network, change and therefore separate from and betray the others. For the individual, they constitute both *controlling others* (rulers) and, especially, *significant others* (friends) and, let us not forget, sexual partners and – even more important – *affective partners* (lovers and loved).

So, in the final analysis, although we take rationality as a starting point, we arrive at the conclusion that the affective element must not be forgotten. Although we consider the individual, we highlight the network as an important system of relations, more than simply a source of norms and rules. Although we start from the hypothesis that there are many networks available to the individual, we demonstrate the fragility of this plurality.

The Macrosocial Dimension: Collective Discourse

We may turn to a directly macrosocial viewpoint to interpret the role of norms instead of the micro or medium level ones used before. Guizzardi, Stella and Remy (Chapter 9) share this view to a degree, although they suggest following a dual analytical pathway consisting of both the macro and the medium level. At the macro level, they suggest the importance of the concept of society as a *collective arena*, denote the process for the creation of collective norms of behaviour as being one of negotiation, and state that the object of the negotiations-transactions are 'behaviours, but especially, symbols and consensus'.

The result is not a construction of norms as such, but a construction of a collective discourse. This is a dynamic process which occurs among various and different collective agents. The main groups among them are scientists and producers of scientific knowledge, organizations responsible for health policies, groups of experts and technicians (jurists, economists, scholars of bio-ethics, communication experts), politicians, churches and religious organizations. They negotiate with each other from different positions of power, and therefore their ability to impose their own themes and solutions within the discourse also differ.

In this model the accent is placed on a collective construction of a representation of the AIDS problem, by means of a social discourse whose content is multiple, complex, not necessarily consistent, changeable and at different levels. This collective discourse has at least four contents:

- definitions of reality;
- identity;
- morality (and therefore of the norms);
- authority.

The site where they exist and are visible is the media system. The media take part in the process also as social agents in their own right, especially since they have become the constructors of the conditions that decide what is real and what is sayable about AIDS.

The result is the creation of representations of the situation, in which different parts are played by actors who act out the situation on stage, including what is to be done, how to place oneself in the various roles of the play and, most of all, how to decode this particular situation. Here the microsocial level comes into play, since the perception of the situation represented at a collective level and the relative norms are re-elaborated at the level of the individual and the reference group. Thus we have, on the one hand, a reconstruction of meanings and, on the other, the elaboration of collective strategies and collective norms of small groups for processing the complexity.

The model is a circular one since we need to go back from the network level to the macrosocial one, although the path to do so is far from obvious. It also contains the implicit principle of the relative autonomy of networks, which is probably dual: one toward the macro level and the other toward the individual members of the relational networks.

The Macrosocial Dimension: Changes and Tensions

Using an anthropological approach which draws on Reiss, but differing from him on several points, Deven and Meredith (Chapter 8) put forward a strictly macrosocial interpretation. The concept of script, which replaces for the most part that of norm used so far, is central to their argument. Their functions are defined thus: 'scripts are involved in learning the meaning of internal states, organizing the sequences of specifically sexual acts, decoding novel situations, setting the limits of sexual responses.'

Present-day social change seems to be linked to painful changes in scripts which concern sexual behaviour. This change may be defined as conflictual (although this term is not used by the authors themselves) among large groups in various positions in the community – adults on the one hand (depositories of predominant scripts which are still in use although contested) and young people and homosexuals, on the other. It would thus appear to be a question of a double conflict – a generational one, youth v. adults, and one based on cultural power, the dominant culture v. the weaker ones. The game is played for high stakes – the maintenance or change of codes of conduct which do not regard simply sexuality, but something much deeper, the kinship structure itself. As Deven and Meredith point out, 'both homosexuals and the young are seen as violating a dominant shared sexual script by their respective de-coupling of sex and intimacy.' This viewpoint, therefore, stresses the role of the norm in the maintenance of power and social control. Norms define normality, acceptable behaviour, persons and groups, on the one hand, and abnormality, the persons and groups who are marginalized because of their behaviour, on the other.

Deven and Meredith also touch on an aspect that has already been dealt with by others, namely, the fact that the violation of the norm as a violation of accepted sexual scripts is a source of pleasure, even if they only intend it in the weak sense of psychological reward. This point could be investigated further to see how, in sexuality, the violation of the norm might be a source of pleasure and how the transgression of the norm constitutes a non-marginal component of sexuality itself. The strict enforcement of norms about sexuality and the conflict which always underlies them in society could thus have an internal component, endogenous to sexuality itself. The norm is inevitable not only because it is transgressed but also because the transgression itself is equally inevitable.

Conclusions

We may now be able to provide some answers to the questions raised initially. First and foremost, the number of levels to be considered is three, not two. The first is the macrosocial one, at which norms and responses to the danger are produced. The second is the individual one, where attention is paid to the warnings and the prescriptions are put into practice. The third important level consists of the networks of interpersonal relations.

Though opinions vary as to the significance of this level, there is general consensus on the fundamental importance of the tripartition. Some see a form of circularity among the three levels, while others stress the predominance of the network to such an extent that the other aspects are obscured, but not in fact eliminated. If anything, the problems to do with the macrosocial level have yet to be fully explored; the macrosocial dynamics seems rather to be taken for granted and deserve more detailed attention. On this point, the role of the media is worthy of further study. The media cannot be regarded as mere channels of information or neutral vehicles of collective norms. Rather, the various forms of the media are privileged sites for the production of a complex and dynamic collective discourse.

Another point concerns relations among the levels. There is general agreement on their autonomy. However, considerable effort has been made in these pages to show the relativity of this autonomy and therefore to suggest the elements for an interpretative framework based on this assumption. We are well aware, however, that not all the authors share this view.

The third significant aspect to emerge is that, however one chooses to define it, the overall mechanism is laced with multiple tensions that are by no means always immediately obvious. It is worth recalling the double role of ego and alter within the relational network, the power conflict between generations or cultures, the collective arena where social representations and normative solutions are negotiated, and the individual, who is split between rational choice and the desire to be accepted. What should be stressed is that it is not merely a question of aspects of freedom and control – an inevitable dynamic where norms are concerned. These tensions operate among the different levels identified and the internal elements of each level.

A further point concerns sexuality. Here, those analyses which rely on a rational-type paradigm as well as those based simply on conflictuality reveal their limitations, since it is inevitable, when one deals with the affective sphere, that factors which underlie the principle of contradiction will come to the fore. The temptation is to use only those factors, for example, behavioural ones, that appear more scientific, since they adhere to the principle of non-contradiction and are certainly more reassuring. Though opinions differ, one thing, however, is clear. The efforts of both theorists and researchers must converge if we are to overcome this limitation.

References

PRYOR, J.B. and REEDER, G.D. (Eds) (1993) *The Social Psychology of HIV Infection,* Hillsdale NJ: Erlbaum.

GERRARD, M., GIBBONS, F.X., WARNER, T.D. and SMITH, G.E. (1993) 'Perceived vulnerability to HIV infection and AIDS preventive behavior: A critical review of the evidence', in PRYOR, J.B. and REEDER, G.D. (Eds) *The Social Psychology of HIV Infection,* Hillsdale NJ: Erlbaum, pp. 59–84.

Chapter 13

New Conceptual Perspectives and Prevention

Dominique Hausser

Introduction: Setting the Stage

The first AIDS cases were identified in June 1981. Although impressive gains have been made in our scientific knowledge of the AIDS virus since its discovery in 1983, no effective vaccine has been discovered. There is no treatment that can prevent the disease's eventual fatal outcome. Although great progress has been made in treating the associated opportunistic diseases, preventing the transmission of HIV is currently and will continue to be for many years the only way to control this epidemic.

The mechanisms of HIV transmission are known to be limited to transmission through exchanges of blood or blood products, transmission through sexual relations, and mother-to-child transmission during pregnancy, delivery and breast-feeding. Except for mother-to-child transmission during pregnancy, the ways to avoid HIV transmission have been known since early in the epidemic, yet the epidemic is far from under control. According to Mann, Tarantola and Netter (1992), between 1992 and 1995 there will be over 5.6 million new HIV infections. The largest number of new HIV infections is in sub-Saharan Africa, south-east Asia, western Europe, Latin America and North America; the virus is spreading most rapidly in north-east Asia, the south-eastern Mediterranean, south-east Asia, western Europe and eastern Europe.

Although the World Health Organization (WHO) has assisted in the development of national AIDS prevention strategies throughout the world, no single country, apart from Switzerland and the Netherlands, has implemented a clear and consistent national strategy to control AIDS. Switzerland alone has been implementing such a strategy without interruption and conducting a comprehensive, continual assessment of its national strategy. While not national in scope, many countries have implemented HIV/AIDS prevention projects and countless intervention measures have been initiated over the past ten years. For the most part, these programmes have targeted either the general population or populations perceived to be at-risk, such as young people, migrants, male homosexuals, intravenous drug users, and sex workers and their clients.

The majority of these programmes were inspired by the individual-oriented rational or informational perspective exemplified by the Health Belief Model (HBM) and other cognitive utility models as described earlier by Moatti, *et al.* As many authors in this book have detailed, sexual behaviour related to HIV risk has not been adequately explained by these individual-oriented theories and consequently they have lost much of their initial appeal for furthering the mass adoption of safer sex. However, it should be recognized that applied individual-oriented rational models have been moderately successful in raising awareness of the transmission routes of HIV/AIDS and conveying knowledge of some methods of safer sex, particularly condom use. This awareness, while probably necessary, has not been sufficient to change behaviour. One reason is the poor coordination of information campaigns. Despite the widespread use of information programmes, many have not been carried out systematically and KABP (knowledge, attitude, beliefs, and practices) surveys continually indicate that not everyone knows what AIDS is, how it is caught or how to protect oneself from it. Misperceptions about means of transmission persist, and knowledge about safer sex, except condom use, lags far behind knowledge of unsafe sex. Equally important, the information programmes have been quite unsuccessful in transferring a sense of personal risk, a probable prerequisite for action based on information about the severity of AIDS. Another explanation for lack of success that has been given by many authors of the preceding chapters is that individuals do not make sexual decisions alone and communication between partners and amongst peers at any one moment is as important, or more important, an influence on sexual behaviour than any information about HIV and AIDS that an individual has learnt.

What is the reason for the heavy emphasis on information programmes and why don't policymakers and public health authorities usually consider other perspectives? First, perhaps they have limited knowledge of health promotion and prevention method. Second, they are influenced by various ideologies or frames of reference. The next section reviews some of these underlying ideologies that drive HIV/AIDS prevention programmes. The third section of the chapter provides some practical advice for those implementing HIV prevention. In the end we offer a synthesis of how policymakers might use some findings of the different authors of this book.

Dominique Hausser

Ideology and HIV Prevention

Free Market Economy

A tenet of the free market economy and capitalism in general is that individuals make rational choices based on available information. A key function of government is to provide adequate consumer information and foster responsible behaviour. When this mentality is transferred to public health, preventing HIV transmission is often limited to informing individuals about ways of avoiding contamination. It is important to bolster personal responsibility, since only a change in individual behaviour will diminish, even stop, HIV transmission. This line of reasoning serves to move the responsibility of infection from any structural deficits caused by the political and social system to the individual. Social issues related to vulnerability to HIV infection such as poverty, discrimination, lack of access to care and information and drug policy become less central when individuals are assigned the main responsibility for HIV infection.

Morality and power

What is defined as good or bad, what is done or not done or what is said or not said is often the underlying theme of HIV prevention programmes. As Guizzardi, *et al.*, have noted earlier, there is a prevalent public norm against illegal substance use, and sexuality is often a taboo subject. Cohen and Hubert note that the risk reduction philosophy of HIV prevention (safer sex and using clean needles) is often in conflict with powerful, well-established moral authorities such as the church. The Roman Catholic church, personified by the Pope, condemns not only sex outside the bonds of marriage, but living together without the sacrament of marriage. It opposes all 'unnatural' means of contraception, including the use of the condom. For policymakers who believe or at least voice agreement with this system of morality, severe constraints are placed on the types of HIV/AIDS prevention that are possible. They are limited primarily to abstention, monogamy, faithfulness to one's partner and no anal sex. Those outside this moral system are viewed as sinners and, by inference, deserving of what they bring on themselves.

This is in contrast to alternative public health systems that advocate risk reduction such as condom use or clean needles and is relevant for the significant subpopulations that fall outside the strict religious norms. KABP studies have shown that the start of sexual experience usually occurs independently of marriage and there is a world-wide trend to engage in one's first

236

sexual experience at an earlier age. Finally, a large fraction of the population has sex with partners outside a stable relationship. While these patterns vary from one part of the world to the next, apparently most of the world's population engages in risky behaviour or situations and falls outside the moral system prescribed by many church and public officials. The alternative normative system is one that values non-discrimination and a universal right to prevention and care. Evidence of this conflict is often heard in Western culture. The church's view is summed up by the term *innocent victims* which is saved for those who were infected through blood transfusions, during pregnancy, or through sex with a sole partner who did not reveal his or her serostatus. An alternative moral system is encompassed in the phrase *people with AIDS* that is applied to all those infected, irrespective of the route of transmission. Our aim here is not to oppose the normative system defended by the Roman Catholic church in the name of another system. Rather, it is to demonstrate how politically powerful players can introduce a system of constraints on policymakers that makes it impossible to respond to the majority of people falling outside the strict norms of the church.

Biomedical Approach

The biomedical approach to health starts with a belief that human beings are willing to sacrifice everything to live as long as possible. It follows that any behaviour that is likely to endanger life should be prevented. Prevention can take several forms: First, when combined with a belief that an individual is a rational decision maker, one strategy is to inform individuals of the danger of unsafe sex or needle use and for them to take on the responsibility to do everything in their power to resist risky behaviours or placing themselves in harm's way. The advocates of such an approach do not make any allowance for the probability that the event will or will not occur or probability or risk in a specific sexual episode. Second, public health often uses the power of the state to control personal life. Legal bans on dangerous products or behaviours that cause public harm, quarantine, registration and contact tracing are some more frequently used public health measures that often place public health above the open market place, individual rights to privacy or personal freedom of choice. Third, public health campaigns can try to change public norms by promoting the undesirability or desirability of certain behaviours. Last, there is often an attempt to medicalize the problem and find a medical or psychological solution.

Smoking provides a good illustration of these principles. There have been campaigns that provide the medical links to the hazards of smoking. Yet, individuals who are fully aware of the dangers continue to smoke. There have been attempts to ban smoking. The political power wielded by the tobacco industry ensures that tobacco – a product that contains legal psychotropic substances and is clearly linked to fatal health hazards – will not be banned outright. On the contrary, its use has even risen worldwide. Still, successful efforts have been made to regulate its use in different contexts, for example, by limiting its use in offices, in restaurants and on flights. Long-term campaigns to change the public image of smoking have worked in several countries. Some social networks now blacklist or marginalize the smoker, so that smoking becomes intolerable to significant others. This is an effective form of social control. Finally, there is an industry that treats smoking as a medical problem of addiction and looks at the causes of such addiction. An essential component of this approach is to admit that some people derive pleasure from smoking. Even within this stratum of control there is a division between those who suggest that the only effective means of control is to stop the behaviour (abstention) and those whose aim is not to eliminate smoking, but to counter excesses and abusive smoking that lead to addiction.

Quality of Life

This biomedical approach to health often conflicts with the quality of life that individuals and groups seek in their intra- and interpersonal relations. Health is only one element that is necessary for well-being, for quality of life. The needs expressed vary from one person to the next, from one group to the next, and are greatly influenced by the social and cultural norms that reign in the social networks under consideration. Within the social milieu, several factors are essential to well-being, such as working conditions that provide communication with others, housing within a desirable neighbourhood, the availability of training and education and recreational activities with one's family. As Ahlemeyer suggests, another critical factor that is often outside these day-to-day concerns is sexual life quality. He notes that individuals' expectations based on norms or experience will often determine the outcome of their behaviour. A focus on quality-of-life factors suggests that knowing what is important in a relationship is a major determinant of behavioural choices and the function of safer sex in improving quality of life is not simply a matter of prolonging life.

Prevention strategies usually start with an implicit or explicit ideology such as those mentioned above. The strategy is in fact the fruit of negotiation and discussion amongst various partners whose interests and stakes vary greatly. Scientific analysis is only one of the aspects taken into consideration. Information about the virus and the spread of HIV is the start of any prevention programme. How that information is applied to prevention depends on the ideological perspective of the prevention agent. As Guizzardi suggests, the scientist (and we add policymaker) is far from removed from this process of interpretation. Many of the contributors to this book are further concerned about how the messages are received and interpreted. Their primarily theoretical considerations about sexual behaviour suggest why many policymakers who rely on a fixed field of individual-oriented strategies that place the individual at the decision-making peak will not succeed. They suggest various avenues of exploration that are greatly influenced by their own fields. In the next section of this chapter we will examine how different perspectives brought up by the authors might be used by someone who must draw up an HIV/AIDS control strategy.

Reasons Why Existing Models Will Not Work

The contributors to this volume have offered two main types of criticism. The first type is levelled at the models used by most (social) scientists and their simplistic and linear utilization regarding behaviour in general and health-related behaviour in particular. The second type challenges the restrictive description of sexuality, which tends to be equated with pure sex (practices described more or less mechanistically), as if sex could be analysed outside its context and the dynamics that leads to it.

The main criticisms of the individual-oriented utility models and their application are as follows:

1 These models establish linear relationships between knowledge, attitudes and behaviour that are rarely borne out by the empirical data. Even though some authors have tried to render such models more complex by adding various components assumed to change this linearity, such as the locus of control, these models are not applicable because the context of the situation plays a crucial role in behaviour. Sieber (1995) showed that using condoms during sex with occasional partners was hardly a given for all men and women. The proportion of people who always use condoms rose between the first and third interviews in their study, in line with the national data (Dubois-Arber, *et al.*, 1994; Hausser, *et al.*, 1991), but the behaviour of two-thirds of the people studied (some 100 seronegative individuals recruited at an anonymous screening centre) varied over time. They protected themselves a certain amount of time, then no longer protected themselves, then resumed protective measures. All possible combinations of changing to safer sex, changing to unsafe sex, and sticking consistently to safer or unsafe behaviour were seen. Van Druten and Van Giessen, *et al.* (1994) also found that the sex practices (penetration/no penetration, insertive/receptive/both) of each member of a cohort of male homosexuals varied over time. What this suggests is that

the type of situation or, to use Alhemeyer's term, *intimate system* makes a great difference in the type of sexual behaviour. The challenge is understanding the context and interaction that produce different types of sexual behaviour.

2 Standardized questionnaires usually do not enable collection of sufficient parameters, particularly interaction-oriented and contextual factors, to permit analysis of sexual decisions. As Ingham and van Zessen and Moatti, *et al.*, pointed out in earlier chapters, the tendency to focus on the risk of infection and the immediate causes of the infection has led investigators to aim their questions at their interviewees' sexual practices and neglect the contextual elements that can explain the behaviour. Although the larger European surveys (those carried out in Switzerland, France, Belgium, and Great Britain) include questions about the respondents' sex partner or partners, such questions permit only limited analysis of the dynamics of the partners' relationship. When only demographic and structural variables are used to predict sexual behaviour and the risk of HIV infection, the results are often presented as the probability that one group is more likely than another to contribute to a given behaviour. This amounts to an epidemiological analysis of sexuality in which researchers search for a culprit as they look for the cause of a disease. More current analysis has explored the complexity of partner relations and how the context of the relationship are important elements in a sexual decision (Marquet, Hubert and Peto, 1994).

3 Most individual-oriented utility models are static and often the operationalization of the predictor and outcome variable are not independent. In addition, there is frequently an assumption that correlational analysis between static and individual level characteristics and sexual behaviour is causal. As suggested by systems models and as detailed by Cohen and Hubert in this book, sexual behaviour is highly conditional on the time in a person's life when it occurs and on the context of the situation. To indicate the limited nature of the operationalizations, Ingham and van Zessen claimed that none of the 14 behaviour change models described by King and Wright used more than seven of the 20 or so variables they extracted from all the models. Perhaps more importantly, the way researchers have operationalized and interpreted concepts such as risk perception and the social dimensions is problematic.

In addition to these criticisms of the individual-oriented utility models, several contributors to this volume highlight the difficulty of describing, understanding and analysing sexuality. The main problems they underscore are as follows:

1 In HIV/AIDS prevention sexual behaviour is often linked to health or illness. In reality, as noted by Bastard, *et al.*, sexual relations are

perceived above all in connection with pleasure and intimacy. A main concern of partners is pleasure. Even when partners think of the possibility of exposure to HIV, the immediate gratification of unprotected sex often outweighs the risk of the less than certain transmission of a virus that will cause illness years later. As shown in examples of interactions presented by Ingham and van Zessen, the considerations that prompt one to use or not use a condom during sex seem to rely on interactional dynamics surrounding intimacy rather than on pre-existing attitudes about HIV transmission.

2   When epidemiological information that ranks type of sex by its risk potential is transposed into prevention information, it does not go over well with its intended targets and usually will not lead to behaviour changes. The sex act is not an isolated incident; it is part of what might be called the sexual episode, which in turn is part of a sexual relationship, that is, an amorous relationship between two people. Several contributors to this book elaborate on this point. In Ahlemeyer's intimate systems the same sexual behaviour has different meaning depending on whether it is part of an intimate, prostitutive, hedonistic or marital system. Ferrand and Snijders discuss how the social network exerts influence on the interpretation of sexual behaviour and how sanctions can work either for or against safer sex. Deven and Meredith, in citing Reiss's works, take a macro-sociological approach to human sexuality and show how vaster societal relations can influence partner relationships.

These different perspectives on sexual behaviour come from different branches of social science, each with its own limitations. They give elements of interpretation that are complementary but sometimes also apparently contradictory. For example, it is not easy to combine the autopoietic aspect of the system and the influence of contextual factors. It is also difficult to distinguish between communication elements and the actors' status within a system. What is more, there is a likelihood that this explanation will become quite complex because each partner may be involved in several systems that may be part of a network of systems that themselves make up a system. This confronts us with the limits of being able to validate an explanatory model that would encompass all the components of each intimate system on the basis of empirical findings.

3   The context of a relationship and the meaning of sexual intercourse change over time. Surveys take one, or at best a few still pictures, but sexual behaviour is part of a continuous movie. The meaning of the same sexual act will change over time as different partners and contexts are introduced into the picture. The temporal perspective, which was analysed in particular by Cohen and Hubert but also stressed by Moatti, *et al.*, Ingham and van Zessen and Bastard, *et al.*, is often rightly considered a confusing variable in the various models examined in

this volume. Cohen and Hubert look at time from an intergenerational, intragenerational, individual or interactive level and each level has several dimensions that must be considered. The interactions between the various levels cause rapid, constant change in the situation. For example, the situation of a 15-year-old today is not identical to that of a 15-year-old ten years ago. The AIDS epidemic has changed, and so has knowledge. To take another example, the situation of a 15-year-old who has sex for the first time will not be identical to that of a divorced person starting a sexual relationship with a new steady partner.

4   The limitations of the instruments available to social scientists and the link between the subject under investigation and the investigator have prompted the contributors to this volume not to propose explanatory models; they are even less inclined to propose predictive models in the usual sense of the word. Several authors in this book, including Bastard, *et al.*, Guizzardi, Ferrand and Snijders, Ahlemeyer and Ludwig and Ingham and van Zessen, try to describe constellations or typologies in which the risk of HIV transmission is one of the components of, rather than an effect of, various variables. All of the authors are adamant about focusing on the relationship's dynamics, the interaction between sexual partners and the context in which the relationship takes place, instead of the individuals. This suggests an approach to prevention where partners become involved in understanding better their own behaviour in various situations and redefining their sexual behaviour to allow for HIV risk.

Practical Implications

Before concluding, I feel it is worthwhile to underline a few specific suggestions that follow from the texts written by the various contributors to this volume.

1   Prevention messages must be customized to specific populations at risk and within certain contexts that place persons at risk of HIV infection. It is important that the messages be widely distributed and no one be left out; and there should be a systematic effort to involve different target populations, such as young people and homosexuals, as part of the prevention efforts. Given that individuals belong to several different social networks, prevention messages should be consistent, even if they are given in quite different forms. Some young homosexuals might be thrown off balance if they received different messages through different channels aimed at one or the other group (Guizzardi, *et al.*, Cohen and Hubert, Moatti, *et al.*, Ahlemeyer and Ludwig), in which case these young homosexuals would be more

likely to ignore both types of information, even to feel that they were not directly concerned. Some findings indicate that even if consistent messages are sent out they may be perceived differently. This means that prevention messages' forms have to be adapted to target populations; these messages may even be geared toward contextual situations rather than target groups.

2 Rather than being geared to individuals, prevention messages should target social networks with the intent of changing the group norm to safer sex, if it is unsafe sex, or maintaining safer sex if it has already changed. This group norm will address different needs in line with the type of system (Ahlemeyer) and culture (Deven and Meredith) and the situation. Yet, scripts can be constructed within each of these systems and situations to suggest the most appropriate meaning for safer sex as defined by the partners. For example, in one situation it may be a reinforcement of love, in another it could be a means of disease prevention, in another it could be a commitment to family. If the norm is changed completely, however, people will simply use a condom without reflecting on the reasons why it is used.

3 The AIDS epidemic is not external to the building of a relationship. Each stage of the epidemic brings with it different knowledge, community commitment to fight against AIDS, types of concerns and interactions among partners, and different perceptions of personal threat (see Cohen and Hubert, Chapter 11). The epidemic contributes to the relationship's construction of sexual behaviour to the extent that each person is concerned by AIDS, social norms are modified by AIDS, and the AIDS epidemic influences individual and group behaviour (Bastard and Cardia-Vonèche, Cohen and Hubert). On a macrolevel, despite the degree of individual involvement or whether AIDS is taken consciously into account, the AIDS epidemic effects sexual relationships, parent-child relationships, and social networks.

4 AIDS prevention is a very long-term undertaking. Young people enter the sexually active cohort every day, and it is probably easier to introduce safer sexual values to partners just beginning sex than to change the values of those who have established sexual patterns and are entrenched in their sexual systems. Young people's relationship skills and knowledge and attitudes are what will determine the prevalence and incidence of HIV over the course of the pandemic.

Conclusions

Prevention and/or public health officials are currently faced with the need to stop the AIDS epidemic in their communities. This means reducing the new infection rate below a certain threshold level and protecting individuals from the risks of infection. Without being contradictory, these two objectives call for different strategies. The current focus on advocating behaviours that stop the chance of HIV infection might be more effective if it adopted risk reduction strategies that were compatible with the needs and patterns of partner interactions.

To succeed in prevention, it would be useful for policymakers and prevention officials to reflect upon the current assumptions underlying their prevention efforts. Individual-oriented prevention programmes based on the notion of individual responsibility might be supplemented by actively creating situations where partners can engage in less risky behaviours. Messages that have focused on means of transmission might be replaced by those that aim to change group norms and their definition of condom use and safer sex.

The fight against AIDS will not take the same form in 2007 as it did in 1997 or 1987. In ten years' time the AIDS/HIV epidemic and the epidemic of social reactions will have changed. We are facing a pandemic that takes multiple forms but strikes mainly those who are vulnerable due to poverty, discrimination, war and displacement. Policy toward AIDS is not solely in the public health sector. Social programmes that range from reducing poverty, reducing the chance of war, and empowering women to more specific health education strategies that support open communication about sex and sexuality and making condoms and lubricant available each have some impact on the future of the epidemic. Successful HIV-prevention policy will mean coordinating prevention strategies at the societal, individual and interpersonal levels.

The lines of thought laid down in this volume do not offer ready-made solutions. They can, however, trigger new ideas among those who have initiated short-term intervention plans to start medium- and long-term planning and give themselves the means to act upon both the public at large, specific social groups, even individuals. The contributors' different experiences and backgrounds have enabled them to examine the subject from various angles; writing the chapters together has enabled us to find common epistemological threads. The interdisciplinary nature of this undertaking and the interaction of various perspectives has opened for each author new doors to understanding the complex phenomena that are involved in the sexual episode.

Despite the different voices of the authors of this book, one message is voiced in unison. For more successful intervention strategies, it is necessary to move from individual to social and interaction-oriented perspectives. The process of moving from interpersonal-oriented perspectives to practical programmes will require a great deal of conceptual work that includes testing and evaluating new prevention methods and, equally difficult, overcoming an army of resistance that has invested heavily in promoting individual-oriented HIV/AIDS prevention.

References

DUBOIS-ARBER, F., JEANNIN, A., MEYSTRE-AGUSTONI, G., GRUET, F. and PACCAUD, F. (1994) *Assessment of the AIDS Prevention Policy.* Quatrième rapport de synthèse. Lausanne: Institut universitaire de médecine sociale et préventive (Cachiers de recherche, Document IUMSP 82a).

HAUSSER, D., ZIMMERMAN, E., DUBOIS-ARBER, F. and PACCAUD, F. (1991) *Assessment of the AIDS Prevention Policy in Switzerland.* Troisième rapport de synthèse. Lausanne: Institut universitaire de médecine sociale et préventive (Cahiers de recherche, Document IUMSP 52a).

KING, A.J.C. and WRIGHT, N.P. (1991) 'The design of HIV risk-reduction interventions: An analysis of barriers and facilitators', Report produced for the Global Programme on AIDS (YGP/IDS), World Health Organization, Geneva, by the Social Program Evaluation Group, Queens University, Kingston, Ontario.

MANN, J., TARANTOLA, D.J.M. and NETTER T.W. (1992) *AIDS in the World,* Cambridge, MA: Harvard University Press.

MARQUET, J., HUBERT, M. and PETO, D. (1994) *Comportements sexuels et réactions au risque du sida en Belgique: spécificités bruxelloises. Rapport à la région de Bruxelles-Capitale,* Brussels, Centre d'études sociologiques, Facultés universitaires Saint-Louis.

SIEBER, M. (1995) 'Die Bedeutung des HIV-Tests für die Aids-Prevention', in HAUSSER, D. (Ed.) (in press) *Psychosoziale und kulturelle Aspekte von Aids,* 5, Bern: Verlag Stämpfli A.G.

VAN DRUTEN, H. and VAN GIESSEN (1994) 'Homosexual role behaviour and the spread of HIV'. Paper presented at the Conference *AIDS in Europe,* Berlin.

Glossary

Introduction

This glossary is limited to the general concepts that come up in most of the chapters in this volume. For explanations of concepts that are used by only some of the authors we refer you to those authors' chapters. We cannot claim to give universally acceptable definitions of all the various concepts; we hope merely to clarify the meaning or meanings that they have most often in this book. When the same concept is used with different meanings in line with the authors' different theoretical perspectives, we have likewise taken these differences into account.

Actancial explanation

Type of explanation in which a phenomenon (such as HIV/AIDS risk-related behaviour) results from the individual's or *social actor*'s own decisions, actions and interactions, in which the individual or social actor has the power to operate intentionally and independently of the constraints of social structure. English and American sociologists use the term *agency* (Jary and Jary, 1991, p. 10).

Cause

Taken in its broad sense, the cause of a phenomenon, such as sexual behaviour in relation to the AIDS risk, is that which belongs to the phenomenon's constitution. It may just as readily occur at the start of this constitution (e.g., the partners' own pasts and prior knowledge) as that which is anticipated in this process or towards which the process leads (e.g., the partners' expectations and the functions of this behaviour) or be part of the context in which the behaviour takes place, such as the social and normative framework of the partners' relationship or the system of interactions to which the relationship belongs. The cause is the principle of the advent of the phenomenon that the explanation seeks (Ladrière, 1994, p. 250). In the broad meaning chosen here, a causal relationship can take on forms that are far removed from mechanical linear cause-and-effect relationships. For example, they can be systemic, functional, actancial (agency-based), dialectic, or hermeneutic. (See *Explanation*)

Comprehension

In the broad sense, comprehending (understanding) a phenomenon such as AIDS risk-related behaviour consists in reconstituting, in one's thoughts, the processes by means of which this phenomenon arises (Ladrière, 1994, pp. 249–50). Each theoretical approach emphasizes specific orders of processes or mechanisms that it considers crucial to understand the phenomenon. For example, the culture's influence, the normative pressures exerted by the network of significant others, the significance of the relationship for the partners, the dynamics of the relationship itself, and the balance of power between the partners. The form that this effort to understand takes in scientific work is the explanation. (See *Explanation*)

In line with W. Dilthey and M. Weber's school of thought, understanding or comprehending (*verstehen*) consists in revealing the meanings that the actors attach to phenomena through a methodology of interpretation. It thus is the opposite of the causal explanation of phenomena (*erklären*).

In this book the word *comprehension* or *comprehending* is usually used in its broadest sense.

Dialectical explanation

In a dialectical explanation, all social systems are characterized by a continuous process of contradictions between its elements and resolution of these contradictions. Any and all phenomena are moments in this dialectic process and must thus be explained by their positions in this process. This dialectic point of view may be applied to the knowledge production process itself. Indeed, the need to resolve the contradictions between speculative theories and between such theorizing and real-world experiences is the springboard of advances in knowledge (Franck, 1994).

Explanation

In its broad sense, explaining a phenomenon consists in relating the phenomenon to a context, a trend, or other phenomena in order to comprehend the phenomenon. The act of taking a phenomenon out of isolation makes the phenomenon comprehensible (Ladrière, 1994, p. 250). The explanation for a phenomenon can take a wide variety of forms, even combine several of them. It can give priority to system effects (systemic explanation), to the functions of the elements of the whole (functional explanation), to the dynamics of the actual relations between *social actors* (actancial or agency explanation), to the contradictions between components of a whole (dialectic explanation), to the meaning of the experience (hermeneutic explanation), etc. (See *Comprehension, Cause*)

In W. Dilthey and M. Weber's school of thought, some authors contrast explaining (*erklären*) and comprehending (*verstehen*). Explaining a phenomenon such as behaviour thus consists in establishing the causal relations from which it results, whereas comprehending consists in elucidating the meanings that the actors attach to the phenomenon by means of a methodology of interpretation.

In this book the word *explanation* is used mainly in its broad sense. *Causal explanation* and *comprehension* in the narrow sense then become two of the various forms of explanation.

Factor

Any element that contributes to explaining a phenomenon. It is generally used in this book as a synonym for cause. (See *Cause*)

Functional explanation

A type of explanation whereby any feature (such as behaviour) of a social system (such as the relationship between sexual partners) is explained by its contribution (or function) to the system's self-reproduction. According to the functional explanation, the specific functions that are carried out by the system's components are dictated by the needs of the whole system.

Hermeneutic explanation

A type of explanation characterized by the search for the significance of human behaviour and action. The hermeneutic explanation consists in revealing a *signified* from a *signifier.* For example, not using a condom during sex (signifier) may signify the partners' mutual attachment (signified).

Institution

A standardized, generalized, and socially widely accepted set of norms organizing an area of life in society (examples: marriage, monogamy, education, etc.). By extension, all social practices and representations that have such characteristics (examples: homophobia, romantic love, etc.). The word *institution* is often used to speak about concrete organizations (the State, a hospital, the media, an association, etc.) when one wants to underline their institutional functions and dimensions. Institutions fulfil the functions of socialization, social control and regulation.

Interaction

Generally speaking, an actor A (an individual or group of individuals) interacts with an actor B when A's behaviour *vis-à-vis* B differs from A's behaviour *vis-à-vis* other actors and the same can be said for B. The two actors act on each other; their behaviour is consequently interdependent. In this book the concept of interaction is used with two different meanings within this general definition. Taken in its narrow sense, the term *interaction* refers to a sequence formed by a precise, limited action or communication by A aimed at B and B's response to A. For example, A suggests using a condom and B refuses. In other cases, the term *interaction* is used with a much broader meaning to encompass all the reciprocal actions and communications that make up a relation involving two or more actors. In this sense, the term *interaction* can be applied just as readily to relations between two sexual partners, relations within a social network, relations between partner and their social networks, etc. Depending on one's theoretical perspective, the interaction may be considered a negotiating process, a transaction, a bargaining process, a process of reciprocal strategies within balances of power, etc.

Model

The word *model* is understood here mainly to be the formalization of a theory in an operational system of analysis that includes a set of empirical hypotheses from which it is possible to deduce a set of consequences that are directly connected to the phenomenon under study (example: Health Belief Model) (Boudon and Bourricaud, 1986, p. 388).

The term *model* is occasionally used, however, with other meanings, such as a conception of the individual or society (for example: the rational individual model), norms of conduct, etc.

Norm

A standard, rule or set of instructions that is specific to a group or society and the function of which is to regulate its members' behaviour. In theory, there are no norms without social control and the threat of punishment. However, the concept of the norm varies greatly in line with one's theoretical perspective. For example, some authors make a distinction between effective or actual norms, which the individual generally abides by because they are accompanied by social control, and ideal or stated norms, the functions of which are basically symbolic for the reference social group. (See *Institution*)

Rationality

In the more general sense, *rationality* is choosing the appropriate means to achieve objectives. An individual or actor is said to be rational if he compares the relative efficiency of different available means with regard to an end and sometimes the ends themselves in order to maximize his benefits.

Safer sex

Behaviour that tends to reduce the likelihood of sexually transmitted infection, e.g. using a condom, having sex without penetration etc.

Sexual relationship

The various episodes of sexual intercourse involving two or more partners but also all the interactions and acts of communication that lead to, frame, and give meaning to the partners' sexual intercourse.

Social actor

Individual or group that interacts with other individuals or groups that engage in social actions, i.e., actions aimed at other actors. (See *Interaction*)

Social control

The set of practices by means of which a social group enforces or encourages conformity amongst its members, or among others, and their compliance with its norms. (See *Norm*)

Social network

The set of an individual's social (family, professional, social, etc.) relations. The social network is both a resource for the individual, who can mobilize it in line with his/her objectives, and an important source of social control over the individual.

Socialization

The process of transmitting and internalizing culture, especially social norms.

Structure and structural explanation

In a very broad sense, any arrangement of elements forming a specific configuration. Structural theory considers all phenomena to be elements of a structure that have to be explained by their positions in their structure. More specifically, in the social sciences a structural explanation sees society and its components (institutions, subgroups, etc.) as structured systems that determine individuals' behaviour. This perspective is often contrasted with that of agency (Jary and Jary, 1991, p. 636). (See *Actancial explanation*)

Systemic explanation

A type of explanation that is usually considered to have the following characteristics:

- Reciprocal causality between the interacting components. The components behave differently than in other relationships; otherwise their behaviour would be independent from the relationship being considered.
- The parts being arranged in a special configuration.
- Self-organization, which leads to (the system's) conservation and relatively closed boundaries.
- The constant transformation of relationships amongst the components according to internal laws where the system's conservation is ensured by the constant transformation of its internal relations.
- A hierarchy of levels from the most complex to the simplest.

(Berthelot, 1993; Franck, 1994)

Theory

A structured set of concepts and hypotheses (the latter being ties between the concepts) intended to explain or make a certain order of phenomena, such as AIDS risk-related behaviour, comprehensible.

Main Sources

BERTHELOT, J.-M. (1990) *L'intelligence du social*, Paris: PUF.

BOUDON, R. and BOURRICAUD, F. (1986) *Dictionnaire critique de la socilogie*, Paris: PUF.

FRANKCK, R. (Ed.) (1994) *Faut-il chercher aux causes une raison? L'explication causale dans les sciences humaines*, Paris: Institut interdisciplinaire d'études épistémologiques.

JARY, D. and JARY, J. (1991), *Collins Dictionary of Sociology*, Glasgow: Harper Collins.

LADRIÈRE, J. (1994) 'La causalité dans les sciences de la nature et dans les sciences humaines', in FRANCK, R. (Ed.) *Faut-il chercher aux causes une raison? L'explication causale dans les sciences humaines*, Paris: Institut interdisciplinaire d'études épistémologiques.

QUIVY, R. and VAN CAMPENHOUDT, L. (1995) *Manuel de recherche en sciences sociales*, Paris: Dunod.

Notes on Contributors

Demosthenes Agrafiotis is professor of sociology at the National School of Public Health in Athens, Greece. He has done research on socio-cultural and psychological aspects of AIDS and sexuality as well as on empowerment of people living with HIV/AIDS. He has published articles on the social perception of AIDS and AIDS as a socio-cultural phenomenon, including 'Cultural Unfoldings' (1983), 'Cultural Discontinuities' (1987), 'Health and Illness, Socio-cultural Dimensions' (1988) and 'Mobile Image' (1992), all in Greek.

Heinrich W. Ahlemeyer is a sociologist and head of the Institute for Systemic Social Research (ISYS), a non-profit research organization at Münster, Germany. He has done research in areas such as organization, prevention and the sociology of sexuality. His study of the communicative properties of social movements, *Soziale Bewegungen als Kommunikationssystem*, was published in 1995. A qualitative analysis of the interaction between sex workers and their clients appeared in 1996: *Prostitutive Intimkommunikation Zur Mikrosoziologie Heterosexueller Prostitution.* For his research in the field of intimate communication, he received the Kybernetes 25th Anniversary Award for the most outstanding paper of the Xth International Congress of Systems and Cybernetics at Bucharest, Romania, in August 1996.

Benoît Bastard is a sociologist and senior researcher at France's National Centre for Scientific Research (CNRS). He has been a member of the Paris-based Centre de sociologie des organisations since 1974. His research has concerned the activity of legal professionals and family counsellors, with special emphasis on divorce and the functioning of family and health. He is currently conducting a study of teenagers' health (with Laura Cardia-Vonèche) that will complete the Franco-Swiss study on coping with the risk of AIDS mentioned in this book. Bastard and Cardia-Vonèche have also published a joint volume on premises to allow separated and divorced parents to exercise their visiting rights (*Enfants, parents, séparation,* 1994).

Laura Cardia-Vonèche is a sociologist and researcher at the Institute of Social and Preventive Medicin (Institut de médecine sociale et préventive) of Geneva

University, Switzerland. Cardia-Vonèche has studied the issue of divorce from various angles, including the way it is treated by the judicial system, its economic effects and its consequences for public health. With Benoît Bastard, she published in 1994 *Enfants, parents, séparation,* a volume on premises to allow separated and divorced parents to exercise their visiting rights. She has investigated the dissemination of preventive messages, dietary habits and taking responsibility for health within the family. Currently, she is working with Benoît Bastard on a volume on how individuals cope with the risk of HIV in their relationships and she is conducting, also with Benoît Bastard, a study of the health practices of teenagers and their parents.

Mitchell Cohen is Executive Director of the Partnership for Community Health (New York), an associate at the HIV Center for Clinical and Behavioral Studies, Columbia University, and an associate consultant for the International HIV/AIDS Alliance located in London. He splits his time between developing models for HIV/AIDS prevention and care and providing technical assistance in establishing and evaluating HIV/AIDS prevention and care programmes. He wrote 'Prevention' and coauthored 'Maintenance of HIV Risk Reduction Among Gay Identified Men' in *AIDS in the World* (1992). At the AIDS in Europe Conference in Berlin, 1994, he presented 'The Health Belief Model: Always, Sometimes or Never Useful in Guiding HIV/AIDS Prevention'.

Fred Deven is Head of Unit at the Population and Family Research Centre (C.B.G.S.) in Brussels. He has published articles in Dutch and English on sex education and living arrangements, including 'The Political-administrative Management of School-based Sex Education in twelve European Countries' (1992), and has edited works on the subject: *They really don't know everything! Family life and sex education in Flanders* (1986), *One-parent Families in Europe,* with Cliquet, R.L., (co-editor) (1986) and *Research on 'Reconstituted' Families in Europe* (1996).

Alexis Ferrand is a professor in sociology at the Université des Sciences et Technologies in Lille, France. He is a member of ACSF, the group that conducted the National Survey on Sexual Behaviours in France (1993). After developing research on sociability and friendship, he became interested in analysing the dynamics of elective relationships and the structure of personal networks and published 'Connaissances passagères et vieux amis. Les durées de vie des relations interpersonnelles', in *Revue Suisse de Sociologie* (1989). He is presently studying how sexual relationships are conditioned by partners' other social relations, especially be exchanging confidences. In this area, he has published 'Les modèles relationnels d'échanges de paroles sur la sexualitè' in *Population,* with Mounier, L., (1994) and 'La confidence: des relations au rèseau' in *Sociétés Contemporaines* (1991).

Gustavo Guizzardi is full professor of sociology at the Faculty of Political Sciences of the University of Padua, Italy. His primary interests are cultural change and mass communication studies. He is part of European networks of research on AIDS that include 'EC Concerted Action. The Protocol Development for Comparative Studies on Social and Contextual Aspects of Heterosexual Conduct' and 'EC Concerted Action on Sexual Behaviour and Risk of HIV Infection'. He published several articles about HIV, among them: 'Epidemiological Analysis and the Collective Construction of an Event', in *Mental Health* (1989) and 'The Social Discourse on Aids', in Friedrich, D., Heckmann, W. (Eds), *Aids in Europe. The Behavioral Aspect*, Berlin, (1995).

Dominique Hausser is a physician with a doctorate in public health and prevention. He is currently senior researcher at the Swiss Federal Institute of Technology (IREC/EPEL). He has been working in the AIDS field since 1985. He was successively co-head of the evaluation of the Swiss AIDS prevention policy and director of the National Research Program on Psychological and cultural aspects of AIDS. He is currently working more specifically on accessibility to social and health services of marginalized populations (drug users, migrants, etc.). Apart from many reports on the AIDS prevention assessment, his major publications on behaviours related to health are: 'Campaign against AIDS in Switzerland: evaluation of a nationwide educational programme', in *British Medical Journal* (1987) (with Lehmann, P. *et al.*); 'Towards improved action against AIDS', in *World Health* (1988) (with Dubois-Arber, *et al.*); and 'Does a condom promoting strategy (the Swiss Stop AIDS campaign) modify sexual behavior among adolescents?', in *Pediatrics* (1994) (with Michaud, P.A.). He is also the editor of a series on the psychosocial and cultural aspects of AIDS (by publisher Stämplfi Verlag).

Michel Hubert is a professor in sociology and social sciences research methodology at the Facultés universitaires Saint-Louis in Brussels, Belgium. He was project leader of the EU Concerted Action on Sexual Behaviour and Risk of HIV Infection, under which this book was prepared. He will be main editor of another book arising from the same concerted action, *Sexual Behaviour and HIV/AIDS in Europe*, which will be published by Taylor & Francis in 1997 and focuses on similarities and differences among European countries in behaviour and attitudes towards HIV/AIDS.

Roger Ingham is reader in health and community psychology at the University of Southampton (UK), where he is also Director of the Centre for Sexual Health Research. His interest in sexual health started almost ten years ago when he received an ESRC grant to explore contextual aspects of heterosexual conduct. Since then he has been involved in a range of projects, including work for the World Health Organization, the Health Education Authority and the UK Department of Health. He has recently coordinated a European Commission Concerted Action which involved developing a qualitative research protocol for use in different countries to enable comparative material on heterosexual conduct to be collected. In 1995–96 he was awarded an ESRC Senior Research Fellowship.

Dominique Ludwig (died in 1994) was a research assistant at the Department of Psychology at the Reims University (France), and member of the Social Psychology Laboratory of the Paris Université (V). Her research concerned the psychology of control and the psychology of health, as well as behaviour modification and stress. She was a member of the ACSF group that conducted the National Survey on Sexual Behaviours in France (1993). Her publications in the field of HIV/AIDS include 'Sida, transmission individuelle, revue de question', in *Revue internationale de psychologie sociale*, with Touzard, A. (1990) and 'Analyse de quelques réactions au sida dans une population étudiante', in *Santé publique et maladie à transmission sexuelle*, with Job Spira, N., Spencer, B., Moatti, J.P. and Bouvet, E. (1990).

Philip Meredith is a medical sociologist and head of the patient audit service in the Surgical Audit Unit of the Royal College of Surgeons of England. Previously Deputy Director of the Programme Department in the International Planned Parenthood Federation, his publications inlcude: *Sex Education: Political Issues in Britain and Europe* (1989); *Planned Parenthood in Europe: A Human Rights Perspective*, with Thomas, L. (co-editor), (1986); *Male Involvement in Planned Parenthood: Global Review and Strategies for Programme Development* (1989); and 'Sexology, Sex Education, Contraception and Abortion', in *Handbook of Sexology* (1994).

Jean-Paul Moatti is Director of the 'Epidemiology and Social Sciences Applied to Medical Innovation' Unit of INSERM, (the French publicly funded medical research institute), located at the Paoli-Calmettes Institute in Marseille, France. He is currently a member of the scientific advisory board of ANRS, the French National Agency of Research on AIDS, and has carried out surveys on 'Knowledge, Attitudes, Beliefs and Practices' toward AIDS in France's general population since 1986. Between 1991 and 1994, he was a member of the Steering Committee on 'Social and Behavioural Sciences' of the WHO Global Programme on AIDS. His work on AIDS is related to a more general framework of analysis of human behaviours toward risk and uncertainty presented in his book *Economics of Safety* (1989).

Danièle Peto is research assistant in Sociology at the Facultés universitaires Saint-Louis in Brussels. She is co-author of *Sida: l'amour face à la peur* (with Remy, J., Van Campenhoudt, L. and Hubert, M., 1992) and of 'La relation sexuelle comme transaction sociale: à partir des réactions au risque du sida', in *Vie quotidienne et démocratie. Pour une sociologie de la transaction sociale* (with Van Campenhoudt, L., Remy, J. and Hubert, M., 1994).

Jean Remy is a professor of sociology at the Catholic University of Louvain (UCL) and co-director of the Centre d'Études Sociologiques of the Facultés universitaires Saint-Louis in Brussels. As a specialist in urban life, he is director of the journal *Espaces et sociétés* (Paris) and has written several books and papers on the topic. The most recent one is: *La ville: vers une nouvelle définition* (with Voyé, L., Paris, L'Harmattan, 1993). He is co-author of the book: *Sida: l'amour face à la peur* (with Peto, D., Hubert, M. and Van Campenhoudt, L., Paris, L'Harmattan, 1993).

Tom A.B. Snijders is professor of stochastic models for the social and behavioural sciences at the University of Groningen, in the Netherlands, and a member of the Scientific Board of the Inter-University Centre for Social Science Theory and Methodology. He is especially interested in the integration of statistical modelling with theoretical modelling and is presently active in social network analysis and multi-level research. He has published several papers on these subjects and is now working on statistical methods for monitoring changes in social networks. Some relevant publications are *Estimating hidden populations using snowball sampling*, with Frank, O., (1994) and *Stochastic actor-oriented dynamic network analysis* (1996).

Renato Stella is assistant professor at the Faculty of Political Sciences of the University of Padua, Italy. His main sociological interests are concerned with mass communication research and with the social construction of the body. He has published several articles on the social dimensions of AIDS.

Luc Van Campenhoudt is professor of sociology at the Facultés universitaires Saint-Louis in Brussels, where he is co-director of the Centre d'Études sociologiques. He is also professor at the Catholic University of Louvain (UCL), Belgium. His main publications concern the sociology of education, sociology of deviance, sociology of AIDS and methodology. They inlcude *Manuel de recherche en sciences sociales*, with Quivy, R. (1988); and *Sida: l'amour face à la peur*, with Peto, D., Remy, J. and Hubert, M. (1992).

Gertjan van Zessen is a psychologist and sexologist and is head of the research programme in clinical epidemiology of the recently founded Trimbos Institute of the Netherlands Institute of Mental Health and Addiction (formerly: the Netherlands Institute of Mental Health). Dr. van Zessen has been involved in AIDS research since 1984. Areas of research and publications include three population studies on sexual behaviour and risks of HIV infection among adults and teenagers (1990, 1991, 1995), and quantitative and qualitative studies of prostitutes and their clients, homosexual men, and young adults with multiple heterosexual or bisexual contacts. Together with Dr. R. Ingham (Southampton), he has been coordinating an EC concerted action on cross-national comparative qualitative studies of sexual behaviour and risks.

Index

absolute relevance type 172
abstinence 37, 49, 117, 195, 205, 224, 236
actancial explanations 78, 80–2, 140–1, 182–3, 246, 248
  interaction and risk 65, 67, 68
Africa 154–5, 198, 199, 202, 207, 234
age 7, 92, 105, 110, 120, 170
  see also young people
Agrafiotis, D. 199
  et al. 103, 112, 113
Ahlemeyer, H.W. 3, 4, 25, 40, 80–1, 182, 192–3
  interaction and risk 60–2, 68, 70–1
  and Ludwig, D. 22–43, 77, 128, 131–2, 192, 198, 224–8, 238, 240–3
AIDS Risk Reduction Model (ARRM) 121, 210, 211
anal intercourse 23, 38, 105, 199, 236
anchoring heuristic 115
Asia 155, 202, 234
associative relationships 47–8, 66, 80, 192
attitudes 12, 44, 77, 138, 191
  designing prevention programmes 208, 211
  interactional processes 84, 85–6, 88
  rationality 127–9, 132, 172–3, 174, 176–7
  understanding risk behaviour 100, 103, 106, 118
  see also knowledge, attitudes and beliefs
attribution theory 213

Australia 92, 207
autopoiesis 26, 27, 28, 225, 226, 241
availability heuristic 115

Bandura, A. 90, 112, 208, 213
bargaining 7–8, 9, 71, 186, 192
  see also negotiation
Bastard, B. 5
  and Cardia-Vonèche, L. 48, 77, 79–80, 127–34, 243
  et al. 3, 44–58, 66, 68–71, 73, 77, 81, 130, 140, 182–3, 186, 192–3, 211, 240–2
behaviour change 3, 4, 73, 96, 225
  adapting to risk 44–57
  communication norms 23, 25, 31, 38
  designing prevention programmes 196–7, 206, 208–10, 213–15
  new conceptual perspectives 236, 239, 240, 241
  rationality 127, 133, 164, 176
  social networks 7–8, 9, 19
  understanding risk 100, 101, 104, 107, 112, 121
Belgium 46, 49, 66, 73, 240
Berthelot, J.-M. 61, 69, 183, 252
biomedical approach 237–8
bisexuality 104, 111, 143, 199
Blau, P. 10, 11
  and Schwartz, J.E. 10
blood 103, 206, 234
Boudon, R. 118
  and Bourricaud, F. 77, 250

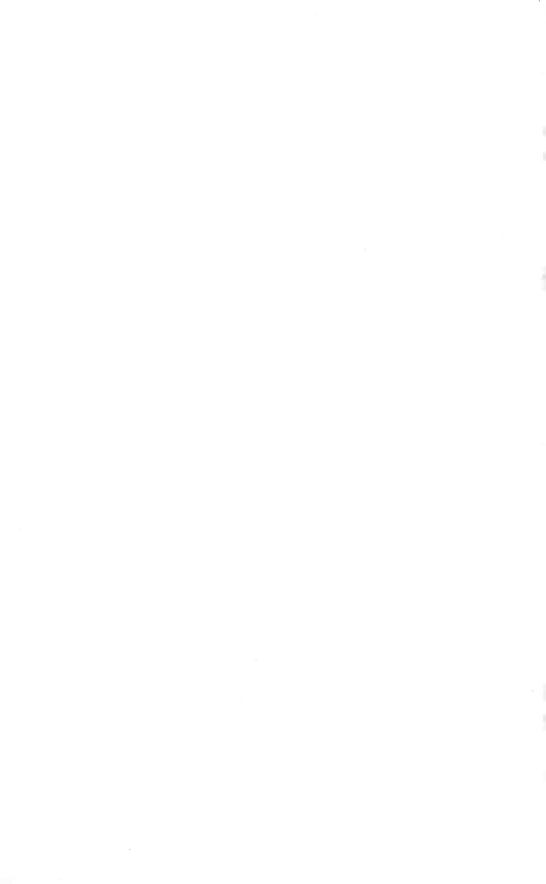

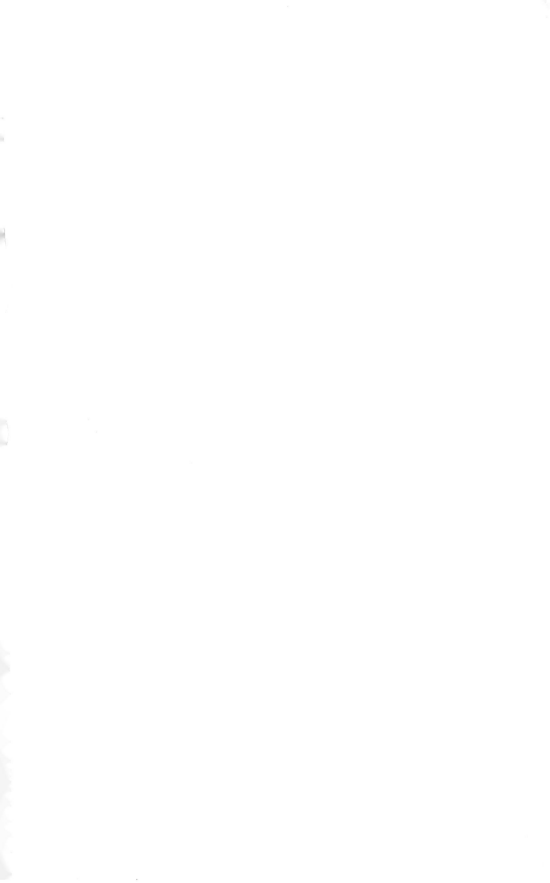

Milton Keynes UK
Ingram Content Group UK Ltd.
UKHW040443071024
449327UK00020B/960